LONNIE

MIX MATCH
MAKE TAKE

COOK WELL
EAT WELL !
&
LIVE WELL !

MIX MATCH

MAKE TAKE

High Energy Food for High Energy People

Daniel J. Witherspoon

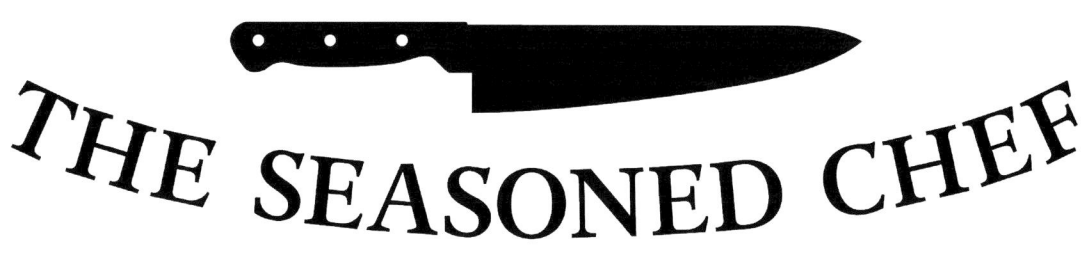

THE SEASONED CHEF

— LEARN·COOK·EAT —

Printed in the United States of America.

ISBN 978-1-943650-81-1

Photographs by Jennifer Olson Photography, Denver, Colorado
www.JenniferOlson.com

Drawing by Cathy Morrison
cathymorrison.blogspot.com

Publisher's Cataloging-in-Publication data
Names: Witherspoon, Daniel J., author.
Title: Mix match make take : high energy food for high energy people / by Daniel J. Witherspoon.
Description: First paperback original edition. | Parker [Colorado] : BookCrafters, 2018.
Identifiers: ISBN 978-1-943650-81-1
Subjects: LCSH: Cooking. | Cooking (Leftovers). | Cooks—United States. | Food—Nutritional aspects.
BISAC: COOKING / Methods / Gourmet.
Classification: LCC TX715 | DDC 641.514–dc22

Published by BookCrafters, Parker, Colorado.
www.bookcrafters.net

In loving memory of my amazing mother
Barbara Jane Witherspoon

And to my noble nonagenarian father
John Eliot Witherspoon
Here's to long life!

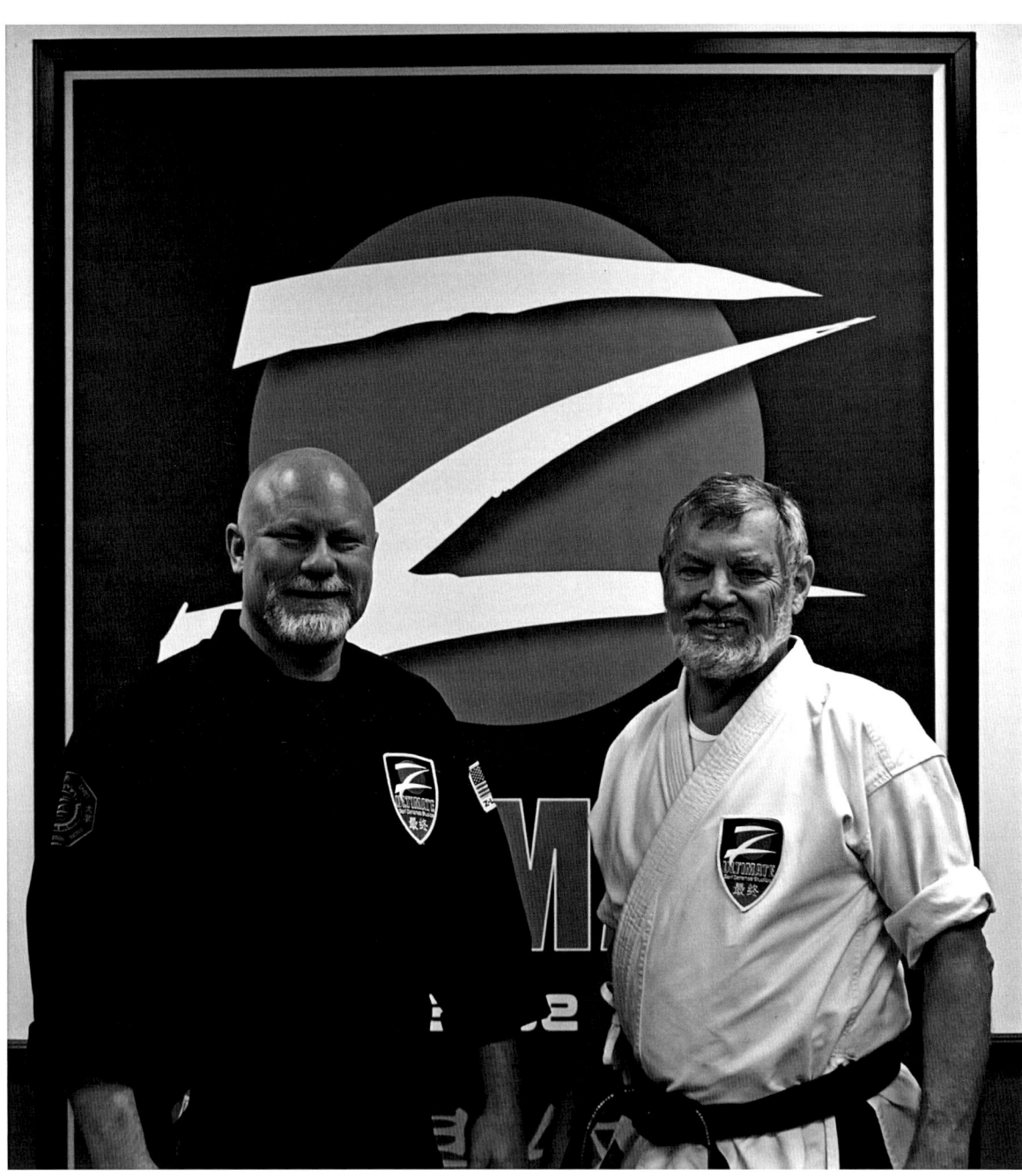

FOREWORD

There are only a few activities in life that we as human beings will do day-in and day-out, every day, for the rest of our lives. Arguably one of the most important of those activities is eating. And, since how we eat and what we eat can significantly affect every aspect of our lives, (our mind, body and spirit) we should learn how to eat healthy and eat well. The challenge: can you make healthy eating taste good without spending hours and hours in the kitchen every day? Yes, you can and Chef Dan will help you do it.

As we all know, life is busy and there are so many daily commitments that lead us to taking shortcuts on healthy eating. Fast food, convenience store snacks, and junk food can easily be a choice because we don't have the time for a restaurant or home style prepared healthy meal. Most of us know we should make better choices but who has the time? But what if making your Sunday dinner can leave you with several gourmet style meals that can easily take the place of those unhealthy alternatives during the week? That was the issue Chef Dan and I discussed over and over. So my question to Chef Dan was simple..."Can you take your amazing, gourmet recipes and create meals that allow anyone to eat for several days without more kitchen time?" His answer was also simple..."Of course I can!" And he did!

I have had the pleasure of working with Chef Dan for many years on cooking skills, team building and healthy eating. His dedication to cooking and helping people cook well using healthy ingredients is akin to any Master at their craft. Just like martial arts training, he brings classical kitchen skills together with practical cooking application. And the results taste delicious.

If you are like me, you're going to be excited to know that you don't have to eat plain and boring food for the rest of your life to be healthy. Chef Dan brings some amazing food options that, and I can tell you, I never considered for a "Make and Take" healthy eating habit. I encourage you to try all the recipes, find your favorites and be healthy and well.

Master William Clark
7th Degree Black Belt
Master Instructor
Z-Ultimate Martial Arts Studios

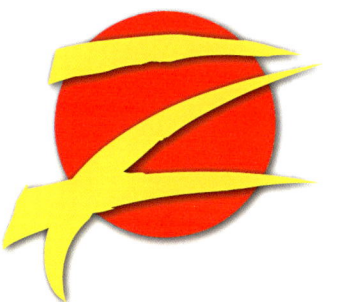

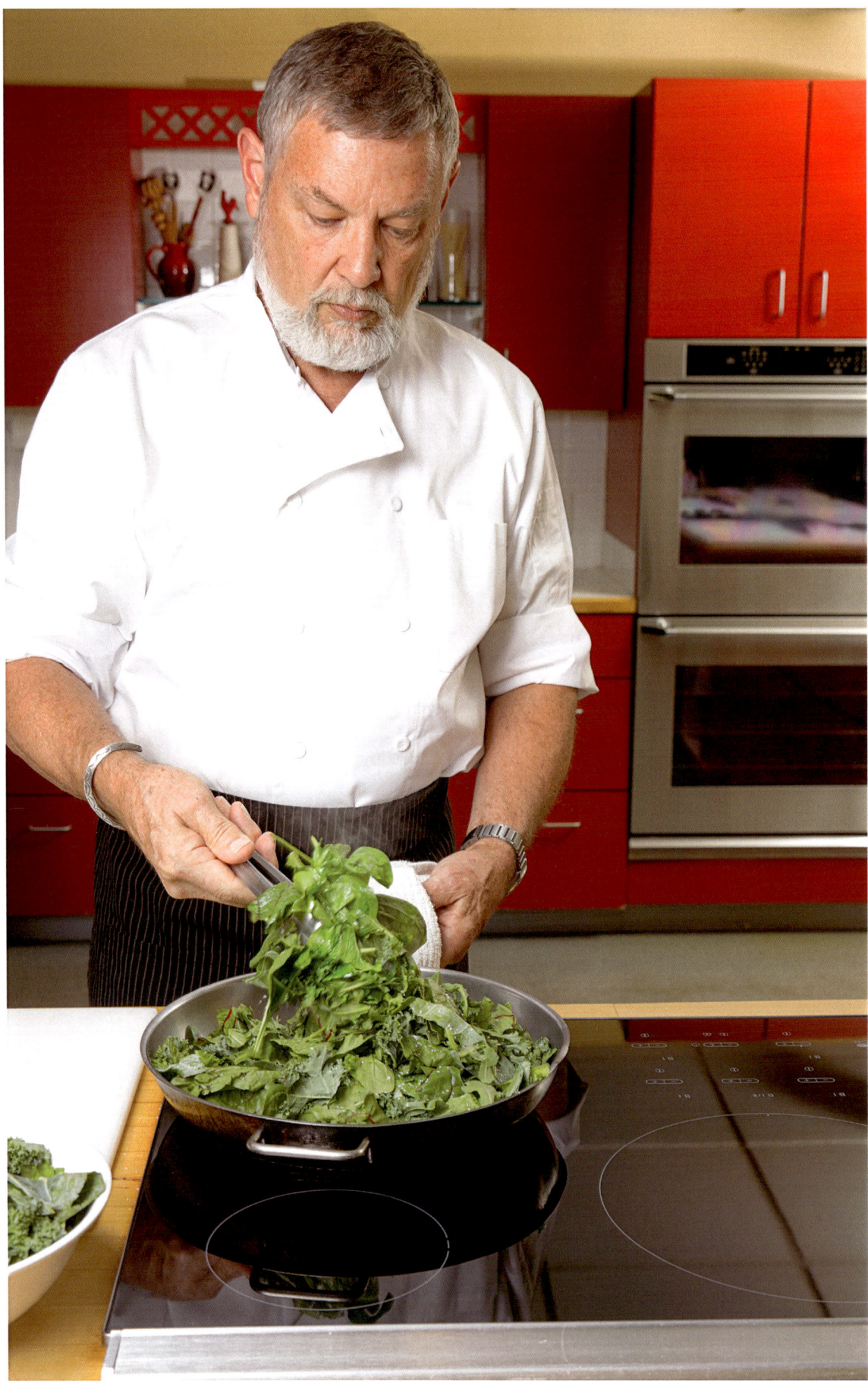

TABLE OF CONTENTS

ASIAN CHICKEN SKEWERS
Tandoori Noodles, 55

MOLE-RUBBED CHICKEN
Grilled Fruit Mojo, Cumin Lime Rice, Grilled Summer Squash, 58

CHICKEN PUTTANESCA
Farro, Spaghetti Squash, 63

PAN ROASTED CHICKEN THIGHS
Curry Coconut Sauce, Steamed Vegetable Medley, Jasmine Rice, 66

ROASTED PORK LOIN
Maple Mustard, Green Beans with Pecans, Baked Sweet Potatoes, 70

SPICE RUBBED PORK TENDERLOIN
Amaranth, Mango Vinaigrette, Lightly Steamed Snow Peas, 74

GRILLED PORK CHOPS
Green Olive Tapenade, Green Lentils, Steamed Carrots, 77

ITALIAN SAUSAGE, BRAISED FENNEL, PEPPERS & ROMA TOMATOES
Hominy Grits, 80

PORK ARRACHERAS
Sweet Potato Pancakes, Grilled Jalapeño Orange Salsa, Crunchy Slaw, 83

GRILLED LAMB CHOPS
New Potato Salad, Grilled Hearts of Romaine, Walnut Pesto, 86

GRILLED SHRIMP BROCHETTES
Parsley Pesto Vinaigrette, Jicama Ensalata, Fresh Roasted Corn, 89

SHRIMP AND VEGETABLE STIR FRY
Steamed Rice, Turmeric Ginger Curry, Tamari, 93

GRILLED SALMON
Gazpacho Sauce, Quinoa Pilaf, Grilled Vegetables, 96

SAUTÉED SALMON
Grilled Pineapple Blueberry Salsa, Edamame with Almonds, 3 Grain Risotto, 100

ARTICHOKE AND CHÈVRE FRITTATA
Baby Red Potato Hash with Fresh Herbs and Garlic, 103

TRAVELING SOUPS, SALADS AND SNACKS

MIX MATCH

PROTEINS
Artichoke and Chèvre Frittata, 103
Asian Chicken Skewers, 55
Sautéed Chicken Breasts, 62
Chili Rubbed Breast of Chicken, 52
Crispy Skin Chicken, 48
Dry Rub Grilled Triangle Tip Steak, 33
Grilled Flatiron Steak, 37
Grilled Lamb Chops, 86
Grilled Pork Chops, 77
Grilled Salmon, 96
Grilled Shrimp Brochettes, 89
Italian Sausage, Braised Fennel, Peppers & Roma Tomatoes, 80
Mole-Rubbed Chicken, 58
Pan Roasted Chicken Thighs, 67
Pan-Seared Flat Iron Steaks, 26
Perfect Roasted Chicken, The, 44
Pork Arracheras, 83
Sautéed Chicken Breasts, 70
Sautéed Salmon, 100
Shrimp and Vegetable Stir Fry, 93
Spice Rubbed Pork Tenderloin, 74
Spicy Bison Meatballs, 41
Triangle Tip Roast, 30

FOUNDATIONS
Amaranth, 74
Baby Red Potato Hash with Fresh Herbs and Garlic, 103
Baked Sweet Potatoes, 70
Brown Rice, 31
Brown Rice with Garlic and Pine Nuts, 49
Creamy Polenta, 52
Cumin Lime Rice, 60
Farro, 63
Fresh Roasted Corn, 91
Green Lentils, 77
Grilled New Potatoes, 33
Hominy Grits, 82
Jasmine Rice, 67
Medley of Roasted Root Vegetables, 46
New Potato Salad, 86
Quinoa Pilaf, 96
Roasted Fingerling Potatoes, 27
Sautéed New Potatoes, 38
Squash Noodles, 41
Steamed Long Grain White Rice, 93
Tandoori Noodles, 55
3 Grain Risotto, 100

VEGETABLES
Bacon Roasted Brussels Sprouts, 27
Buffalo Cauliflower, 131
Cauliflower Fried "Rice", 129
Cauliflower Risotto, 37
Crunchy Slaw, 83
Edamame with Almonds, 101
Green Beans with Pecans, 70
Grilled Hearts of Romaine, 88
Grilled Summer Squash, 61
Grilled Vegetables, 98
Jicama Ensalata, 89
Lightly Steamed Snow Peas, 76
Roasted Asparagus, 34
Roasted Zucchini, 32
Sautéed Leafy Greens, 135
Spaghetti Squash, 64
Steamed Carrots, 79
Steamed Vegetable Medley, 68

FLAVORS
Bacon Mayonnaise, 133
Balsamic Vinaigrette, 29
Black Bean Relish, 52
Black Olive Caper Tapenade, 119
Chili Lime Vinaigrette, 99
Chimichurri Sauce, 28
Citrus Vinaigrette, 79
Curry Coconut Sauce, 66
Gazpacho Sauce, 98
Green Olive Tapenade, 77
Grilled Fruit Mojo, 60
Grilled Jalapeño Orange Salsa, 85
Grilled Pineapple Blueberry Salsa, 100
Lemon Caper Vinaigrette, 116
Mango Vinaigrette, 74
Miso Vinaigrette, 68
Orange Tamarind Vinaigrette, 73
Parsley Pesto Vinaigrette, 91
Roast Vegetable Compote, 47
Roasted Tomato Salsa, 13
Roasted Tomato Vinaigrette, 125
Tomatillo Mole, 31
Tomatillo Salsa, 48
Tomato Pepper Piperade, 41
Turmeric Ginger Curry, 93
Walnut Pesto, 86
Wild Mushroom Salsa, 37

HOW TO USE THIS BOOK

Physical fitness training is easy; a push-up is a simple move. Basic martial arts training is just as easy; an outward block is elementary. Basic cooking skills are easy as well. After all, the technique to properly cook a delicious, juicy steak is straightforward, once you know how. The process of taking these three different skills to a higher level, however, involves commitment, a little discipline and practice. And they are all well worth the effort!

There are no shortcuts or magic pills that can take you to the next level of any skill. Fitness training involves repetition and refinement as well as attention to proper movement. Martial arts is a process of constant learning while teaching the body how to move in a new way, plus gaining flexibility, strength and stamina. The process of cooking has no shortcuts either, but can and should be a lifetime of learning. The art is to tailor basic cooking skills to your personal nutritional goals. And that is where this book is targeted.

Our concept is quite simple. Every healthy meal is constructed of four basic components: a fresh protein, fresh vegetables, flavor (sauce) and a foundation (a whole grain or root vegetable.) We offer recipes that Mix and Match these four components. In addition, we give instruction to Make and Take meals that travel well. Thus, one cooking session can yield several additional meals. This enables high energy people with busy active lives to take control of their diets, and maintain their healthy lifestyle on a convenient day-to-day basis. We have devised fresh, nutritious and delicious meals that can be eaten for dinner on the first day, then adapted slightly the following day with new flavors for variety, or simply reheated and enjoyed again. These recipes are easy to transport in plastic containers or a thermal lunch box, and can easily be packed so they can be popped into a microwave. Portion sizes are really up to you, even though guidelines are given in the recipe. So in other words, eat as much as you like!

You will notice that most of the recipes are quite simple by themselves, particularly the proteins and the vegetables. The beauty of this cookbook concept is in its simplicity. You can eat healthy and delicious foods without spending hours in the kitchen. You will also notice that some of these recipes are very similar to each other. For instance, Grilled Salmon and Sautéed Salmon. But with a slightly altered cooking medium, you achieve a different flavor profile.

These menus, as written, make good solid meals that are well tested. Once you are familiar with this process and the basic idea, you can create a whole new combination of recipes of your own choosing! Just use your extra protein, grain and vegetables with whatever sauce, vinaigrette or salsa takes your fancy that day. The majority of these main recipes (with the exception of those that are to be reheated the next day) can be served on a bed of mixed greens with different raw or cooked vegetables, and a dressing added just before serving. By cooking two recipes at once, you can then interchange the components for the next few days and have even more options.

There are a wide range of foods and recipes not included in this cookbook. Specifically, wheat, refined sugar, and most dairy have been omitted. These ingredients, when eaten in excess, can and will slow the body down. When you're ready to take your physical training seriously, whether in the gym or the dojo, the recipes and cooking styles herein will help you maximize your results.

I encourage you to make a few of the recipes as they are in the Table of Contents. Get a feel for this concept of cooking. Then, switch over to the Mix Match section and begin choosing recipes that appeal to you from the different categories and match those together. Experiment and have fun!

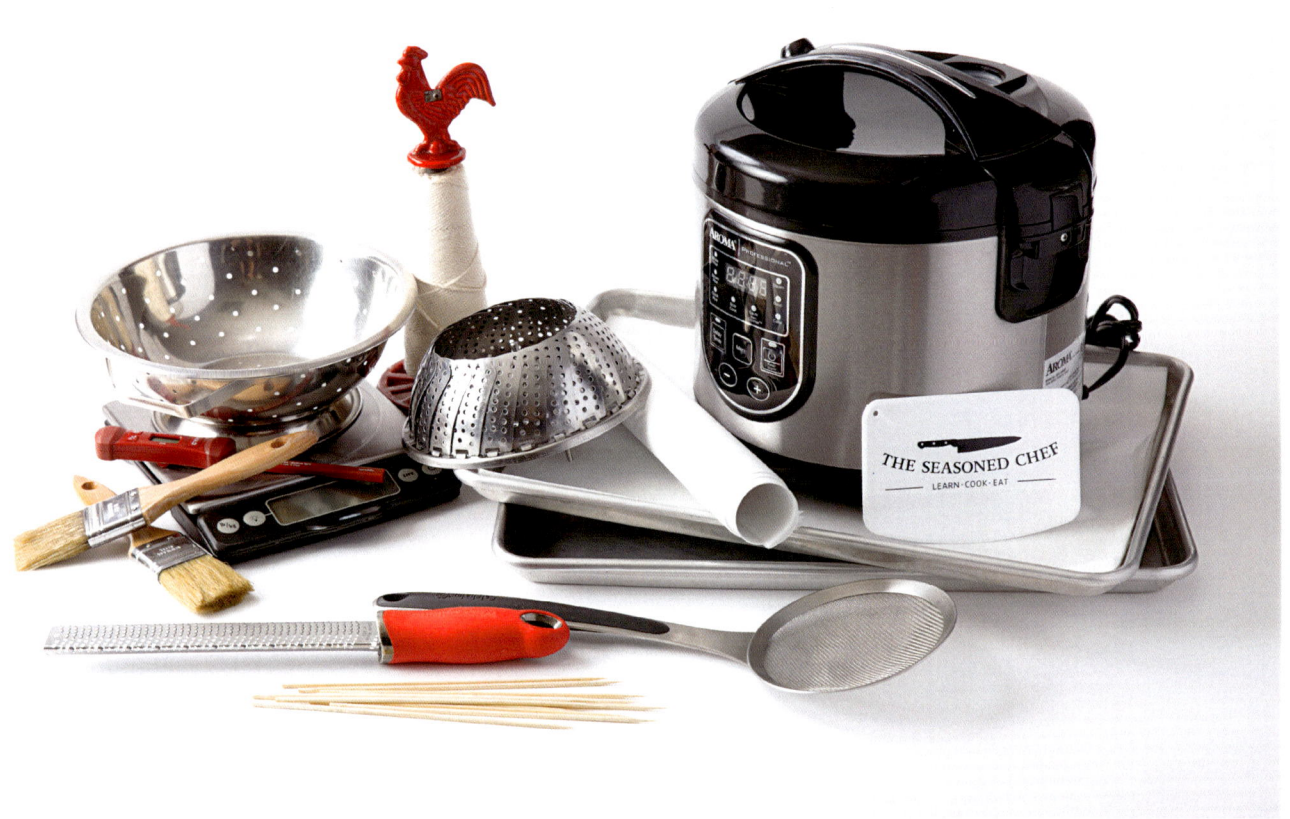

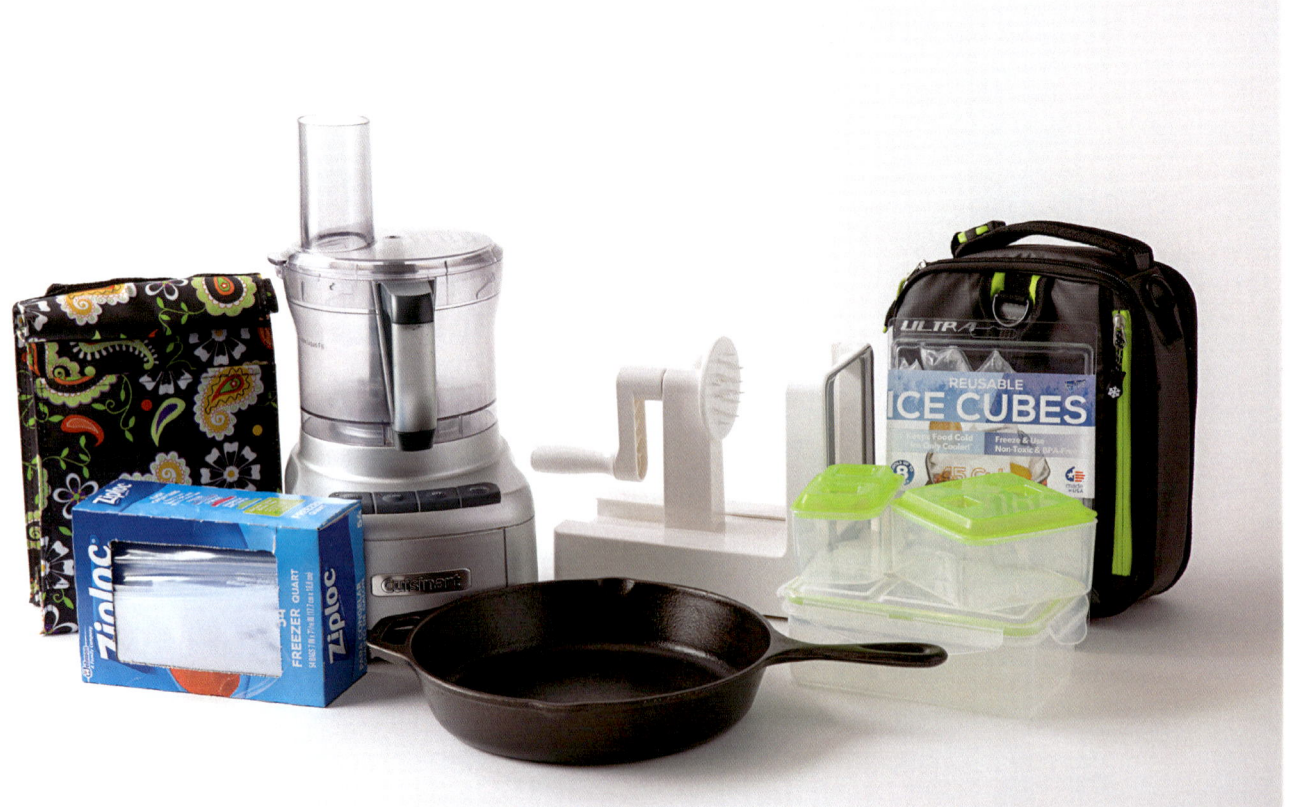

SPECIAL EQUIPMENT ESSENTIALS

Every well-stocked kitchen has the basics: pots, pans, tools, etc. I strongly suggest a few extra specific tools that will help with the recipes in this book. These items are readily found just about anywhere. They are listed in no particular order.

- An insulated, thermal lunch bag or tote
- An assortment of microwave-safe, plastic containers with tight fitting lids
- Self sealing food storage bags
- A digital-read meat thermometer
- An indoor grill plate and/or cast iron skillet
- A digital-read food scale
- A rice cooker
- Bamboo skewers
- A food processor
- A couple of pastry brushes for oiling
- 3-4 rimmed metal sheet pans
- Parchment paper for lining sheet pans
- Microplaner
- A colander
- A sieve
- A bench scraper (This inexpensive plastic tool is priceless for removing cut product from the cutting board safely.)
- A spiralizer
- A steamer basket
- A roasting rack
- Cooking twine
- Reusable ice

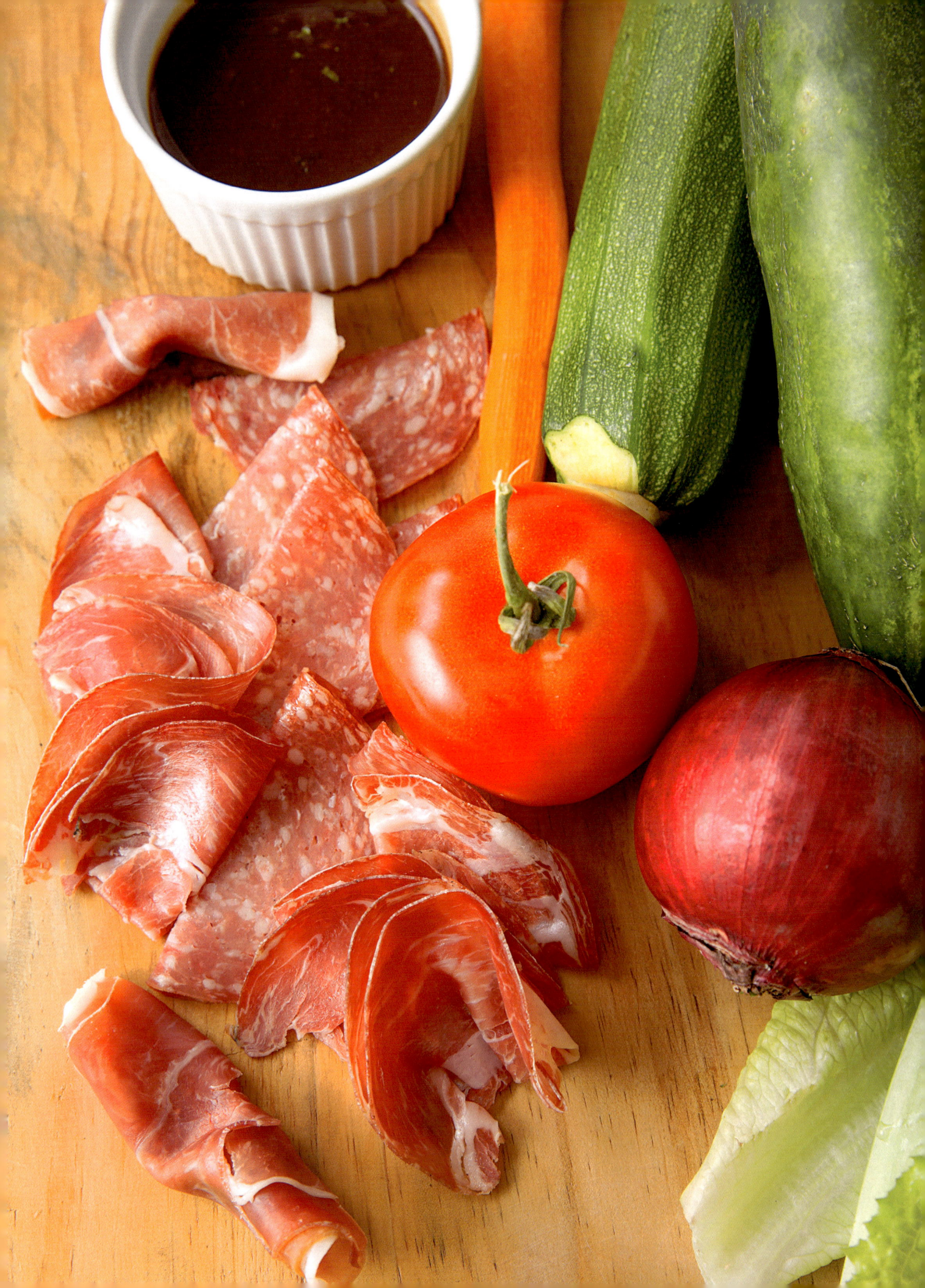

GUIDELINES FOR CONSCIOUS CUISINE

I have been cooking for over 30 years. In my opinion, eating fresh food isn't everything — **it's the only thing!** The best thing you can do for yourself is learn to cook, and by this I don't mean just follow a recipe, I mean learn basic cooking techniques, observe the process, and interconnect those techniques to the process. That will open up your world to a whole new experience — one where fresh ingredients shine, and you develop the confidence to become self-sufficient enough to sustain yourself, your family and your friends for the rest of your life.

Processed food is just a negative food value. There is no need to buy into the industry that produces the enormous supply of packaged "food" available today. Scientific development is out-pacing nutritional analysis, and the world food supply is like the universe — the more you learn, the more you realize you don't know. If you think food consciousness isn't gaining ground at breakneck speed, I challenge you to find a parking space at a natural food store!

Buy *real ingredients* and start educating yourself — for example, limit your refined sugar, white flour and cow's milk intake, don't buy anything that is "low-fat" or "diet" (don't get me started on this....) and expand your repertoire to include ingredients such as vinegars, fresh herbs, olives, sautéed greens, nuts and seeds — fantastic and delicious health benefits all round. If you stick to a varied diet just bursting with fresh vegetables, fruits, meats, fish and whole grains — and start considering "conscious cuisine," as I like to call it, by really *thinking* about your food, by sourcing your ingredients, reading labels, frequenting farmer's markets, and starting to make smart choices — you will be setting yourself up for success for life and putting your health and wellness firmly front and center.

Bon Appetit!
Chef Dan

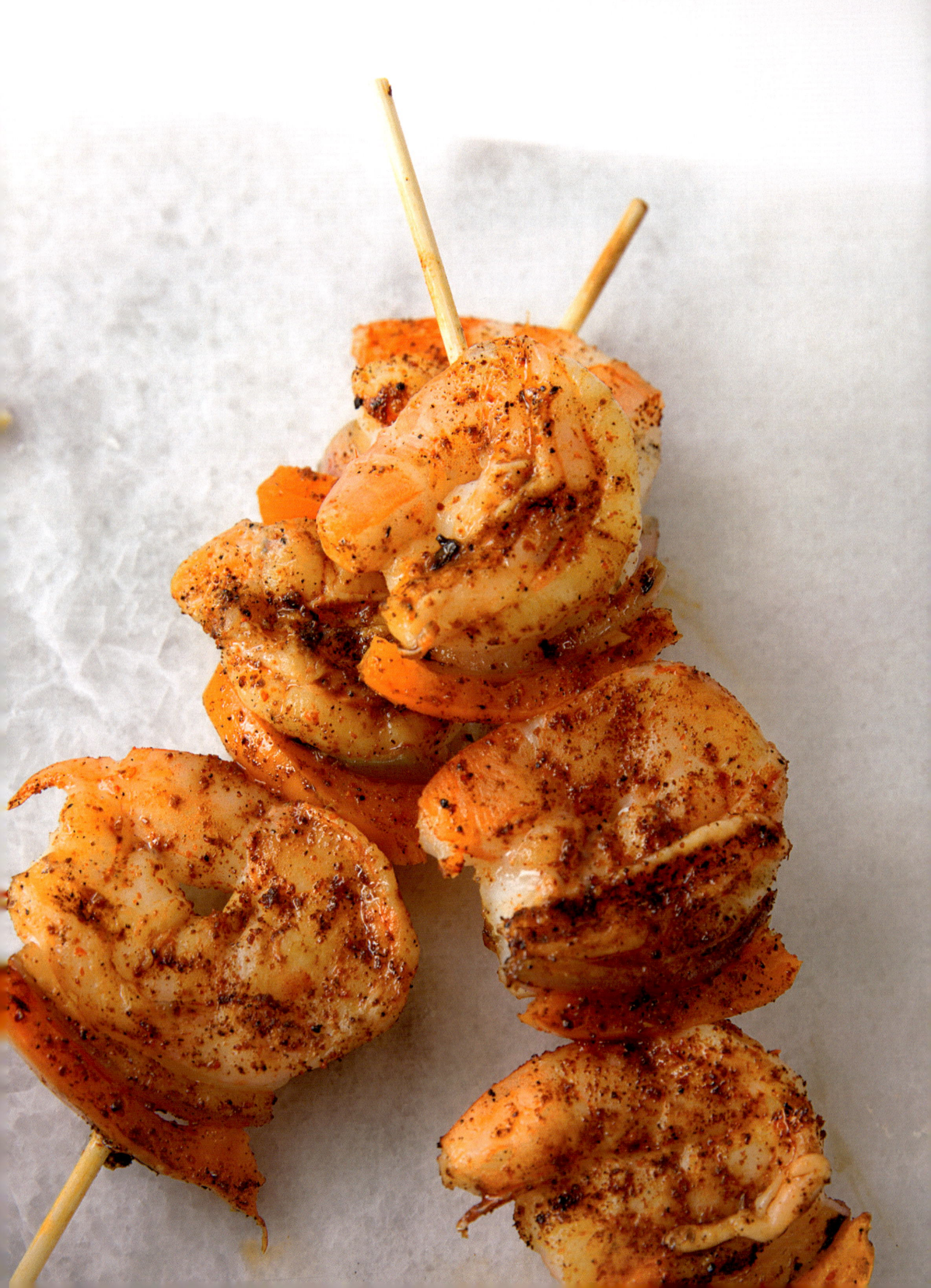

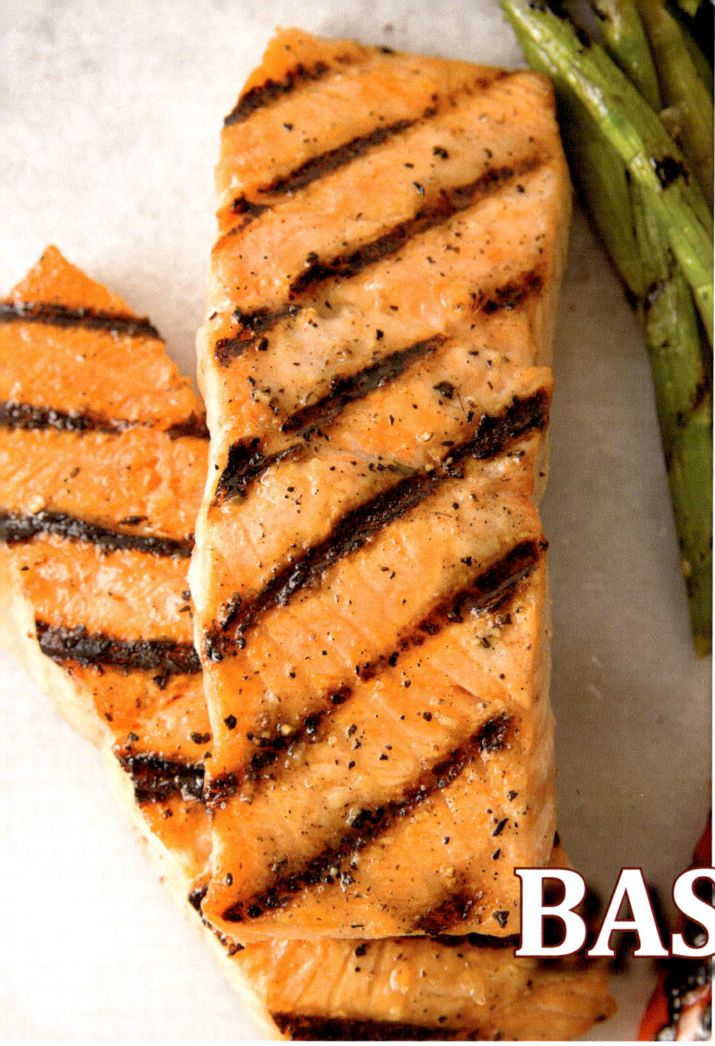

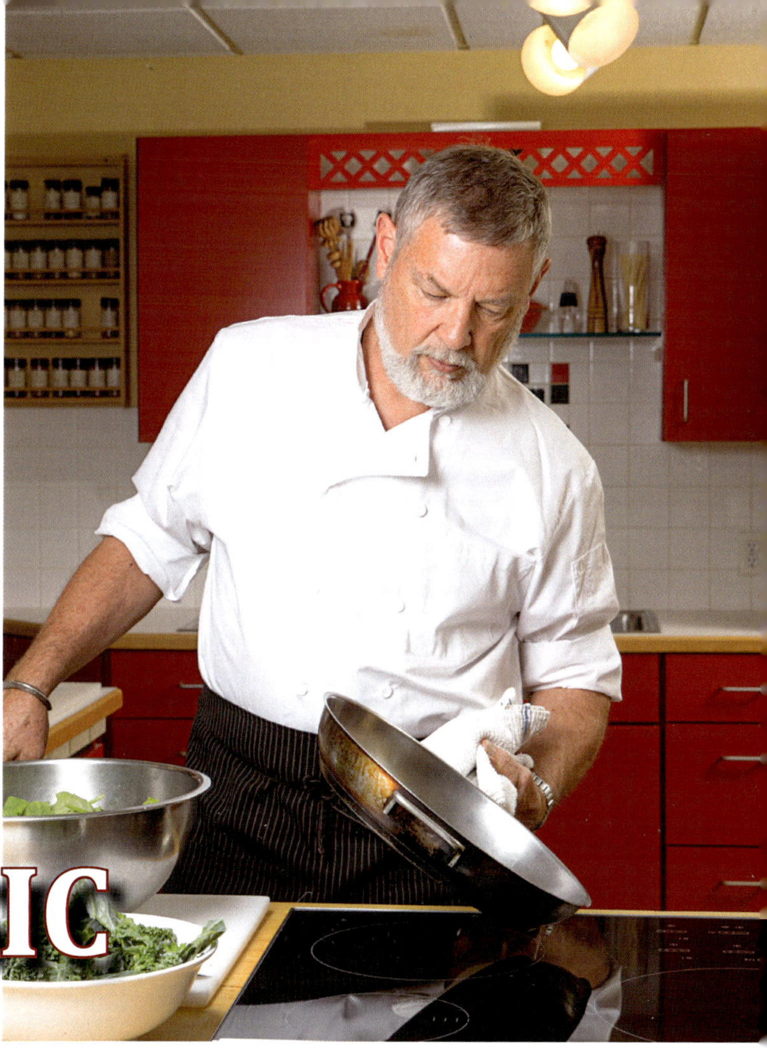

BASIC TECHNIQUES

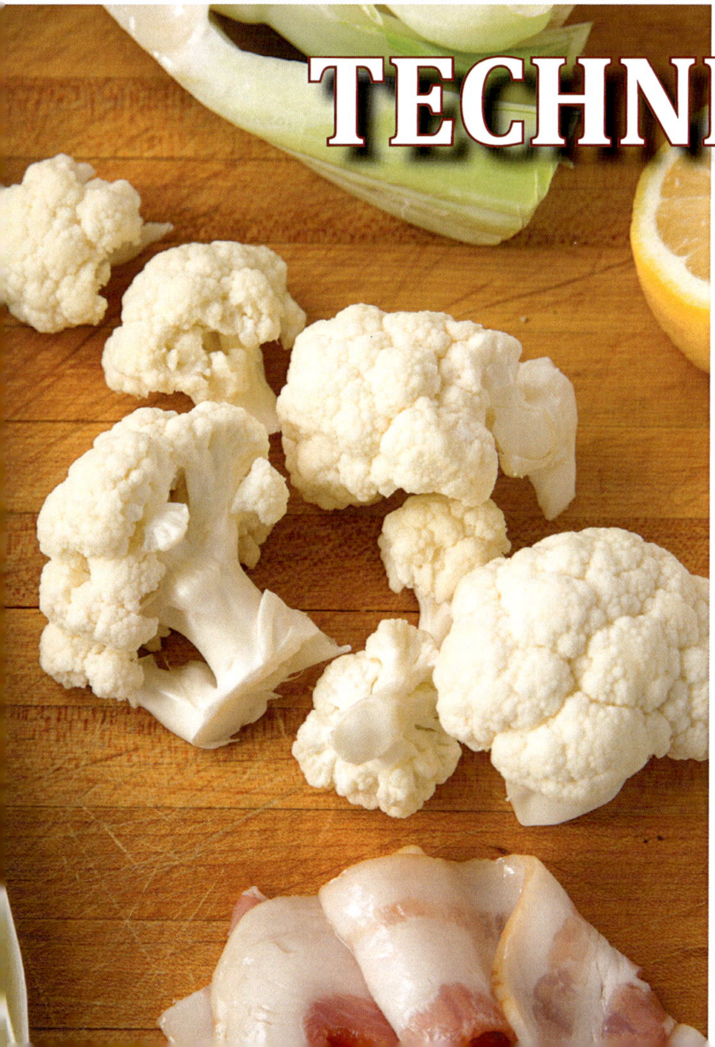

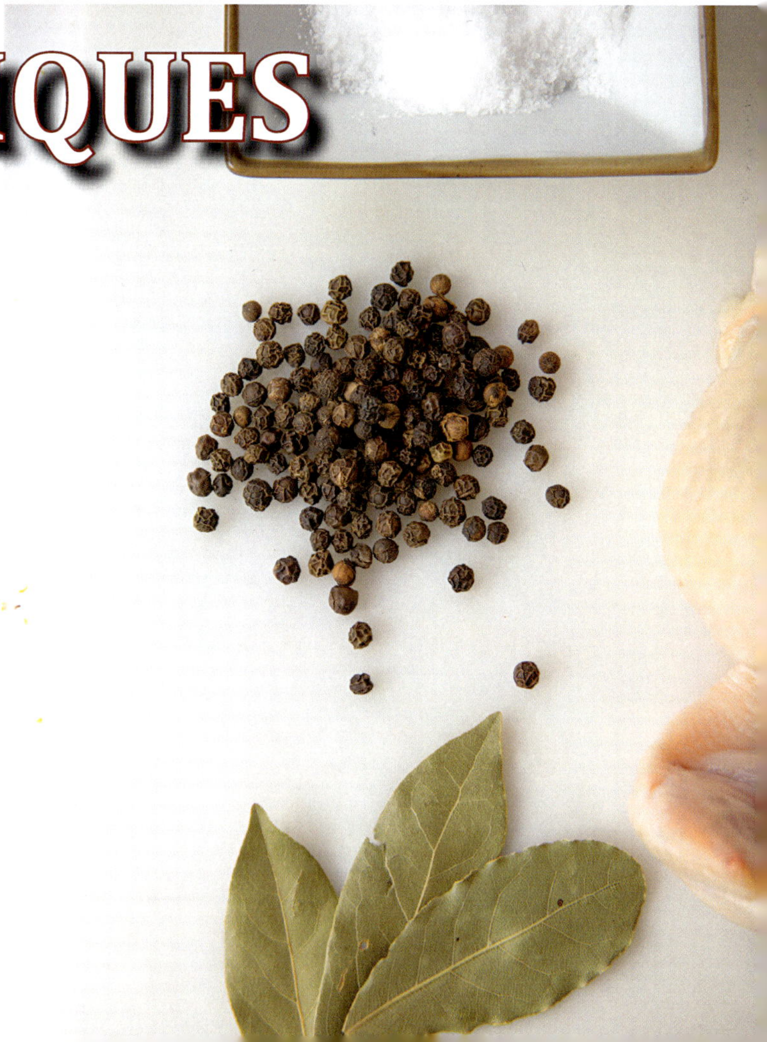

ROASTING PROTEINS

The actual cooking medium, when roasting, is hot air. Whether using gas or electricity, the oven is designed to heat the air inside and thus whatever happens to be in the oven.

Roasting is the preferred cooking method for larger proteins. For example, by using indirect heat, i.e., hot air, a whole chicken can be cooked evenly and thoroughly in an oven without burning the skin or drying out the meat. For larger, tender cuts of meat, roasting allows the tissues and fats to break down gently while the meat itself begins to firm. This allows the fat to infuse the meat with flavor and moisture.

The only battle during roasting occurs when trying to determine the appearance of the outside of the item roasted with the degree of doneness on the inside. A well-browned slightly crisped exterior is generally desired, while a moist, tender, medium-rare to medium center is also highly prized. There are two ways to accomplish these results:

1. For larger roasts, preheat oven to a high temperature (425°F). Place the product in the oven for 15-20 minutes, then lower the heat to a more gentle temperature (325°-350°F) for the duration of the cooking time.
2. For smaller cuts, use a large sauté pan and brown the entire exterior of the item, using sauté techniques over direct heat before placing the item in the oven.

Basic roasting techniques include:

- Always preheat the oven before beginning the cooking process.
- For larger cuts, use a roasting rack or roughly chopped vegetables to elevate the roasted item from the bottom of the pan. This prevents direct heat transfer from the bottom of the roasting pan.
- For smaller cuts, use a pan sized in proportion to the item to be roasted. Too large of a pan will allow the drippings to spread and burn and too small of a pan can result in drippings on the oven floor.
- Lower temperature roasting reduces shrinkage and increases tenderness.
- Whenever possible, allow the item roasted to rest for 5-10 minutes outside of the oven before serving. This promotes tenderness, juicier meat and allows the cooking process to complete.

TEMPERATURE CHART FOR ALL MEATS

Using a meat thermometer, you can use this chart to determine the degree of doneness.

Rare	115-125°F
Medium-Rare	130-135°F
Medium	140-150°F
Medium-Well	155-165°F
Well-Done	170-185°F

Pork should be cooked to an internal temperature of 140-150°F. Chicken breast meat is done when it has reached an internal temperature of 155-160°F. The dark or thigh meat needs to be cooked to an internal temperature of 165-170°F. This poses a problem when roasting a whole bird, therefore it is necessary to determine by personal desire.

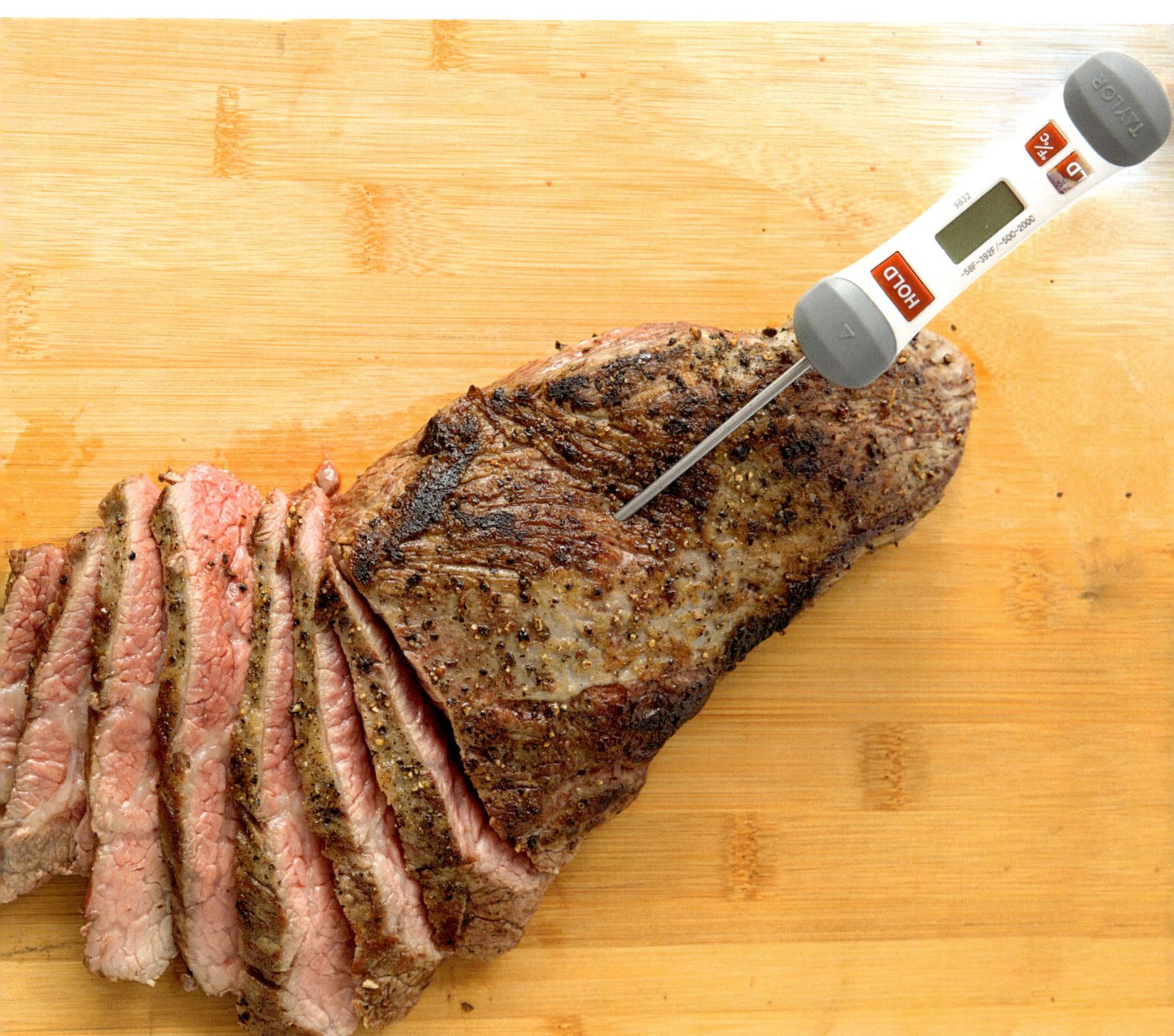

ROASTING VEGETABLES

Roasting is an easy and excellent way to prepare vegetables. This under-used technique has many advantages over other methods. Roasted vegetables can be served alone or combined with other roasted vegetables for a colorful and delicious accompaniment on the plate or buffet. Generally the vegetables are lightly coated with oil and seasoned with salt and pepper prior to roasting. Other dried herbs and seasonings can be added prior to cooking once you have mastered this basic technique.

Some preferred vegetables and their roasting times are as follows. Always preheat oven to 350°F.

Asparagus, medium	6-inch lengths	8 10 minutes
Beets, medium	whole	1-1¼ hours
Bell Peppers	½-inch strips	8-12 minutes
Carrots	split	15-18 minutes
Corn, whole	husked and foiled	12-16 minutes
Eggplant	½-inch thick slices	10-12 minutes
Eggplant, Japanese	split in half	9-11 minutes
Mushrooms*	whole	7-10 minutes

*Some wild mushrooms such as portobellos and criminis are excellent to roast, times varying according to size.

Onions	split in half, skin on	30-35 minutes
Potatoes, Russet	whole	1-1¼ hours
Potatoes, Baby	whole	30-40 minutes
Root Vegetables	¼-inch dice	10-15 minutes
Shallots	whole, unpeeled, covered	15-20 minutes
Winter Squash	split, seeded and diced	15-20 minutes
Yams	whole	40-50 minutes
Zucchini	¼-inch slice	9-12 minutes

Roasting Peppers

This is a good technique for roasting any type of pepper, whether mild or spicy. Preheat broiler to high.

Cut the very top and bottom from the bell pepper. Cut in half vertically and remove the stem, seeds and ribs. Place the two halves on a metal sheet pan skin side up and brush lightly with olive oil. Place under the broiler and cook until most of the skin is blackened. Remove and let cool. When cool enough to handle, peel the skin away from the flesh, being certain to scrape away any black bits of skin with a paring knife.

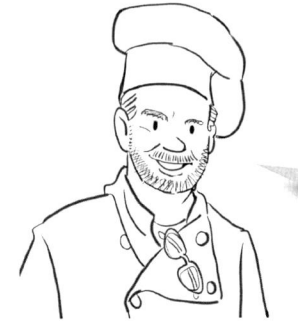

Parchment paper keeps the food from sticking and makes the pan much easier to clean. Use when roasting but not under the broiler!

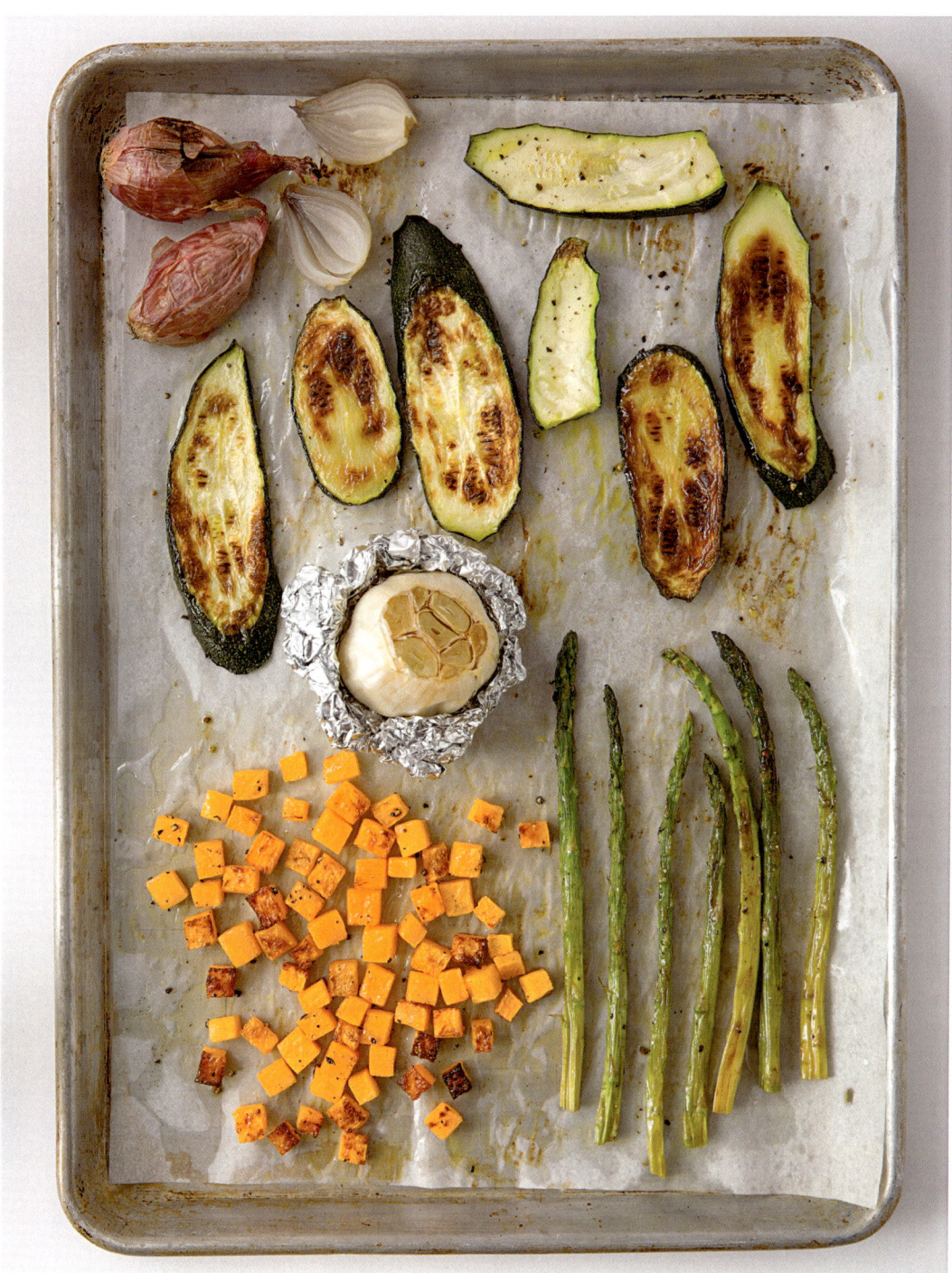

Roasting Garlic

Preheat oven to 350°F.

Remove any loose leaves from the garlic head and cut off the top quarter. Place the head of garlic in a small, thick-bottomed pan and top with 1 teaspoon of olive oil. Cover with a lid or aluminum foil and place in the oven. Cook 35-45 minutes until soft to the touch. Let cool. Squeeze the cloves from the head onto a cutting board and mash and chop finely with a knife until it becomes a paste. Put in a small bowl and set aside until ready to use.

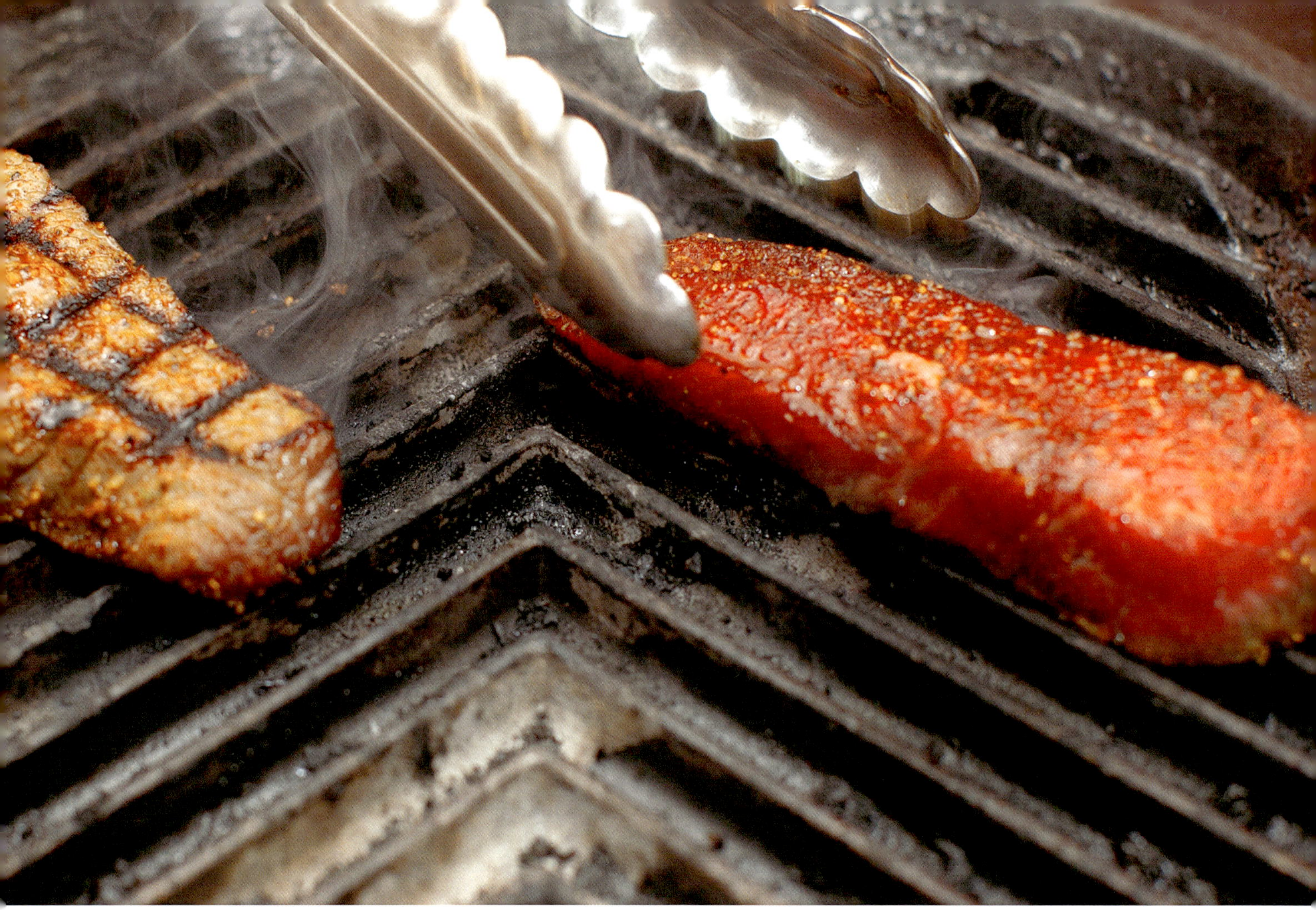

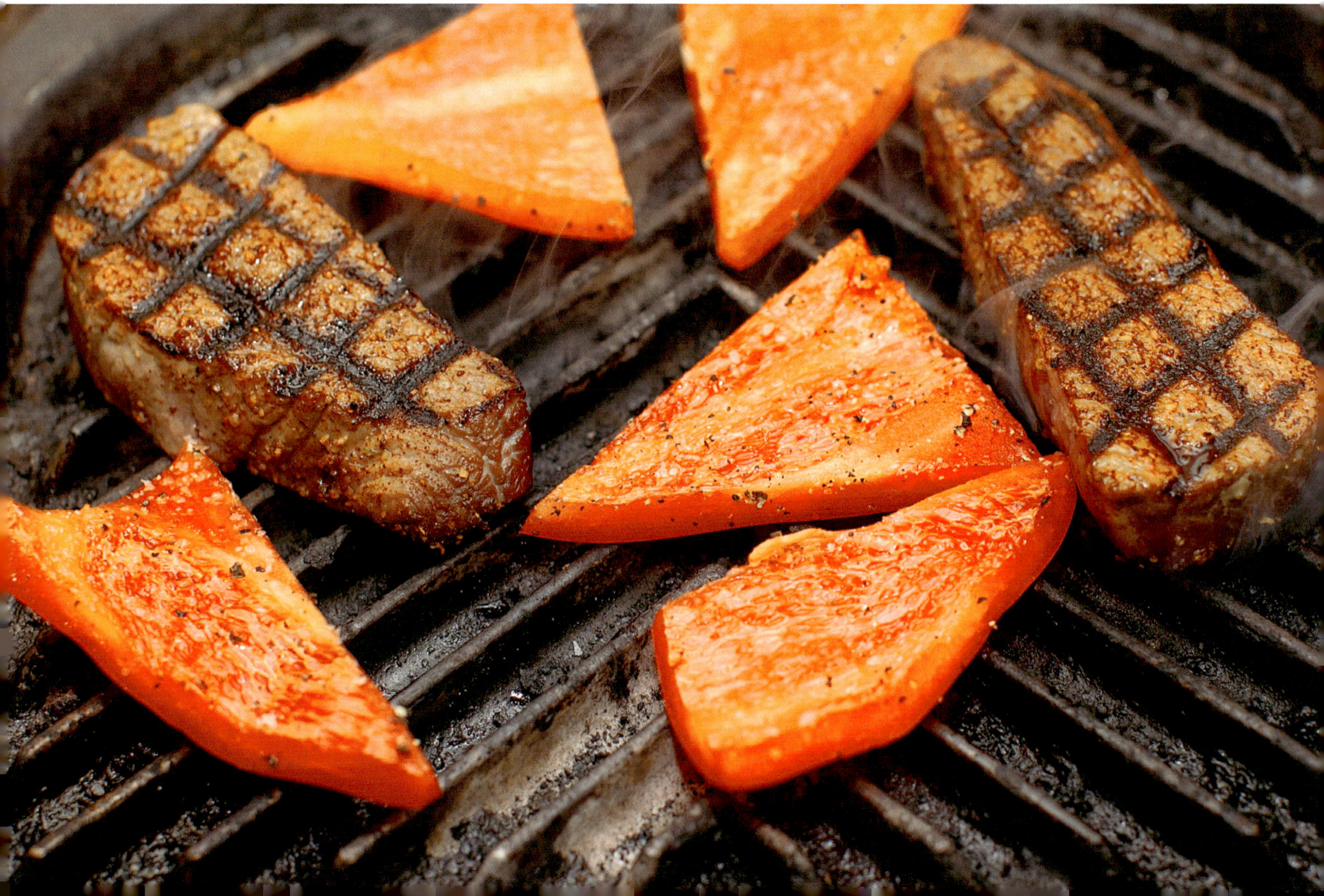

GRILLING TECHNIQUES

Basic grilling involves cooking relatively thin cuts (2 inches or less) of tender proteins directly on a grate, heated by charcoal, gas or electricity at a surface temperature of between 350-650°F. Most basic proteins are cooked on medium high (about 450°F) to high heat.

The actual temperature is irrelevant for the most part, as grilling does not require specific monitoring of the temperature.

The basic set-up rules are:

- Get the grill hot.
- Clean the grill with a good stiff metal brush and wipe with a paper towel.
- Oil the grates lightly. I use paper towels that have been drizzled with cooking oil.
- Whatever the protein or vegetable you are cooking, get it dried, again with paper towels, seasoned, and lightly brushed with oil.
- Use dry seasonings only, like salt, pepper, herbs, spices, or any rub of your choice. If you have used a wet marinade, remove any excess marinade prior to placing on the grill, and then lightly oil the marinated product.
- Place the product on the grates and leave it alone until it is done to your liking, turning over only once when it is halfway cooked.

The cooking time guidelines are:

- Medium rare - 10-12 minutes per inch of thickness, total cooking time.
- Medium - 12-15 minutes per inch of thickness, total cooking time.
- Medium-well - 15-18 minutes per inch of thickness, total cooking time.

For example, a 1-inch thick steak takes about 5-6 minutes on each side.

For internal temperatures, see the temperature chart in Roasting Proteins on page 11.

It's important to remember that most grills have hot-spots on them, so it's worth getting familiar with your grill to know exactly where to place your food so it cooks efficiently.

Although lots of grills on the market are complicated, grilling is simple. There are a lot of accessories available, such as side burners, rotisseries, smoke cooking accessories, beer keg coolers, etc., but these can be a distraction to your basic technique.

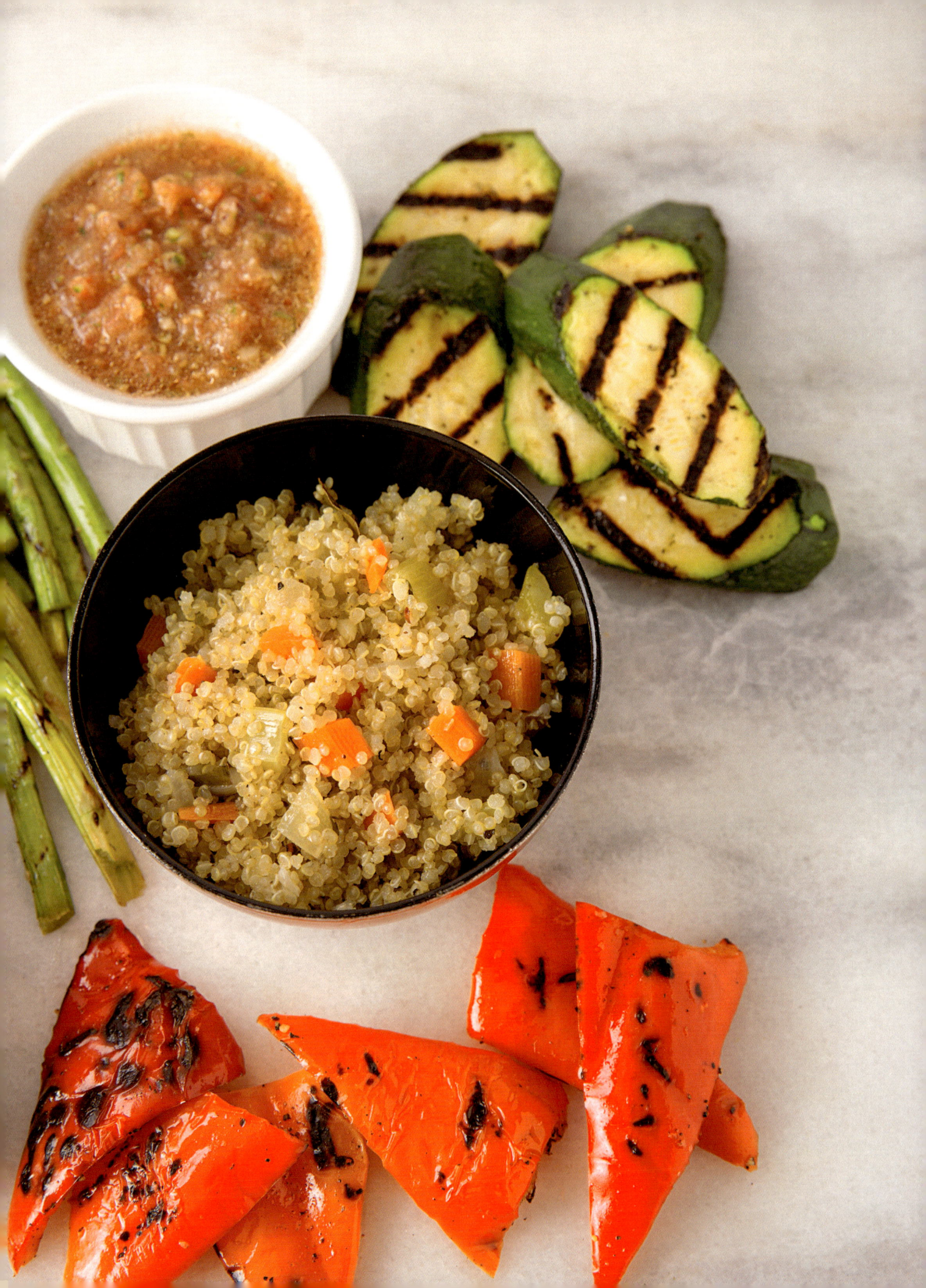

GRAIN COOKING TECHNIQUES

Whole grains are an important part of our daily food regimen. They come in many varieties but the basic cooking technique rarely changes. They are extremely easy to cook when you follow these basic steps:

- Only pre-rinse grain when specifically directed.
- White rice varieties generally take about 20 minutes to cook.
- Brown rice varieties generally take about 40 minutes to cook.
- Wild rice varieties generally take up to 1 hour to cook.
- In general, whole grains take 20-45 minutes to cook with varying amounts of liquid.
- Polenta and grits take 10-20 minutes, depending on the size of the grind.
- Longer cooking times require more cooking liquid.
- Other flavors can be added before or after cooking.
- Some grains need to be stirred, others cannot.
- Some are covered, and some are not covered.

I would recommend buying a rice cooker. They are great for most grains, especially white rice, quinoa, and any other grains that take approximately 15-20 minutes to cook. Some longer cooking grains, however, such as brown basmati rice, might require more liquid than called for on the package directions. Some of my rice cooker experiences have been simple trial and error getting the liquid to grain ratio dialed in. Once you do, this appliance is a reliable convenience.

We usually have a large batch of cooked rice on hand and when we reheat a portion, we often incorporate other flavors like cumin, lime juice, curry powder, etc. to complement whatever entrée we are serving.

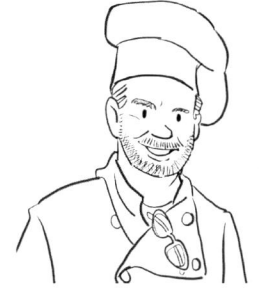

Read each recipe through from start to finish before you begin cooking.

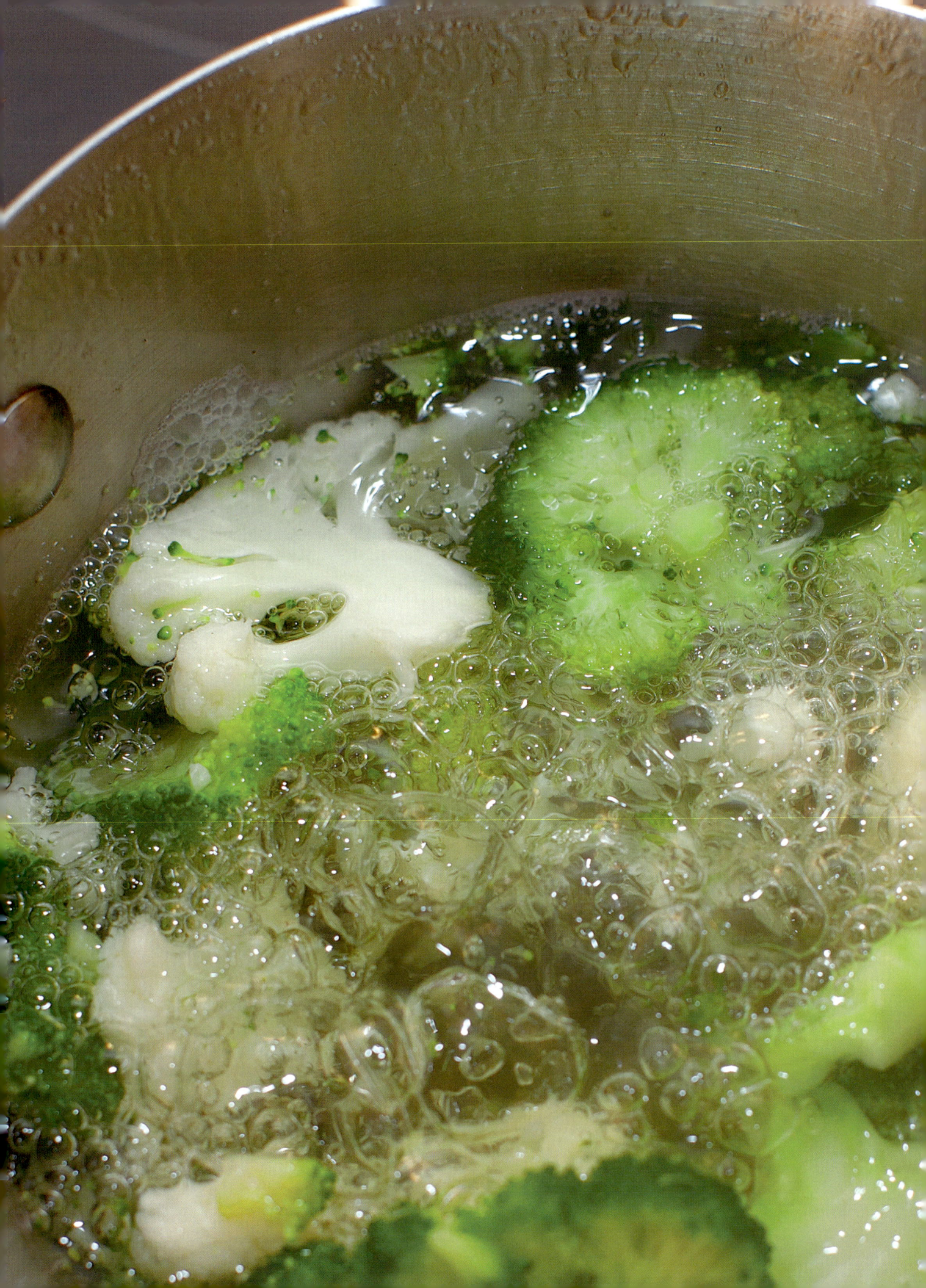

BLANCHING TECHNIQUES

Blanching is a technique that lends itself best to green vegetables and root vegetables. With green vegetables, a relatively large amount of salted water is brought to a boil. The vegetables are added uncovered, and then cooked quickly until just cooked through. They are served immediately or transferred to a container of ice water to stop the cooking process and maintain the color. When cooled, the vegetables are drained and set aside or refrigerated until served.

Root vegetables, having a higher starch content, are started in cold, salted water and brought to a simmer. The duration of the cooking time begins once the simmer stage has been reached. Like green vegetables, they are served immediately or transferred to an ice water bath and drained when cooled.

The ideal way to accurately determine the perfect point of doneness for any vegetable is by using your sense of touch and taste. This skill can be learned quickly with a limited amount of practice.

Cooking times vary between vegetables; however, cooking times are generally considered to begin once the blanching water starts to boil, not before.

The recommended cooking times are:

Artichokes	trimmed	20-25 minutes
Asparagus	5-inch lengths	1-4 minutes, depending on thickness
Beets, medium	whole	30-40 minutes
Broccoli	florets	2-4 minutes
Brussels Sprouts	trimmed	5-10 minutes
Carrots	¼-inch thick slice	5-7 minutes
Cauliflower	florets	3-5 minutes (add Tbsp lemon juice to water)
Corn	whole, husked	2-3 minutes
Green Beans	ends removed	5-10 minutes, depending on season
New Potatoes	whole	20 minutes
Root Vegetables	¼-inch thick	4-5 minutes
Snow Peas	trimmed	20 seconds

NOTE: For steaming vegetables, a smaller amount of water is brought to a boil and a metal basket is fitted into the pot above the water line. The vegetables are added to the basket once the water is boiling, then covered. The cooking times are basically the same and the ice water bath is still essential if not serving immediately.

SAUTÉING TECHNIQUES

Sautéing is a method of cooking proteins with direct heat. It is an efficient way to cook tender cuts of meat and poultry, and all kinds of fish and seafood. Proper sautéing uses small amounts of oil or fat, yet achieves optimal results.

Basic sautéing techniques:

- Always thoroughly dry and season the protein prior to cooking.
- Use a sauté pan that is relative in size to the amount of product to be cooked to ensure that the items are neither crowded nor widely spaced apart.
- Sauté only in a very hot pan with a small amount of oil.
- Do not cover as covering causes steaming.
- Only regulate the heat after the product has been placed in the sauté pan, as cool ingredients reduce the surface temperature of the sauté pan.
- Remember that you can always cook your protein a little more but you can never cook it a little less.

The cooking time guidelines are:

- Medium rare - 10-12 minutes per inch of thickness, total cooking time.
- Medium - 12-15 minutes per inch of thickness, total cooking time.
- Medium-well - 15-18 minutes per inch of thickness, total cooking time.

For example, a 1-inch thick steak takes about 5-6 minutes on each side.

For internal temperatures, see the temperature chart in Roasting Proteins on page 11.

There are few sautéed vegetables in this book because they lose their quality when reheated, and do not travel well.

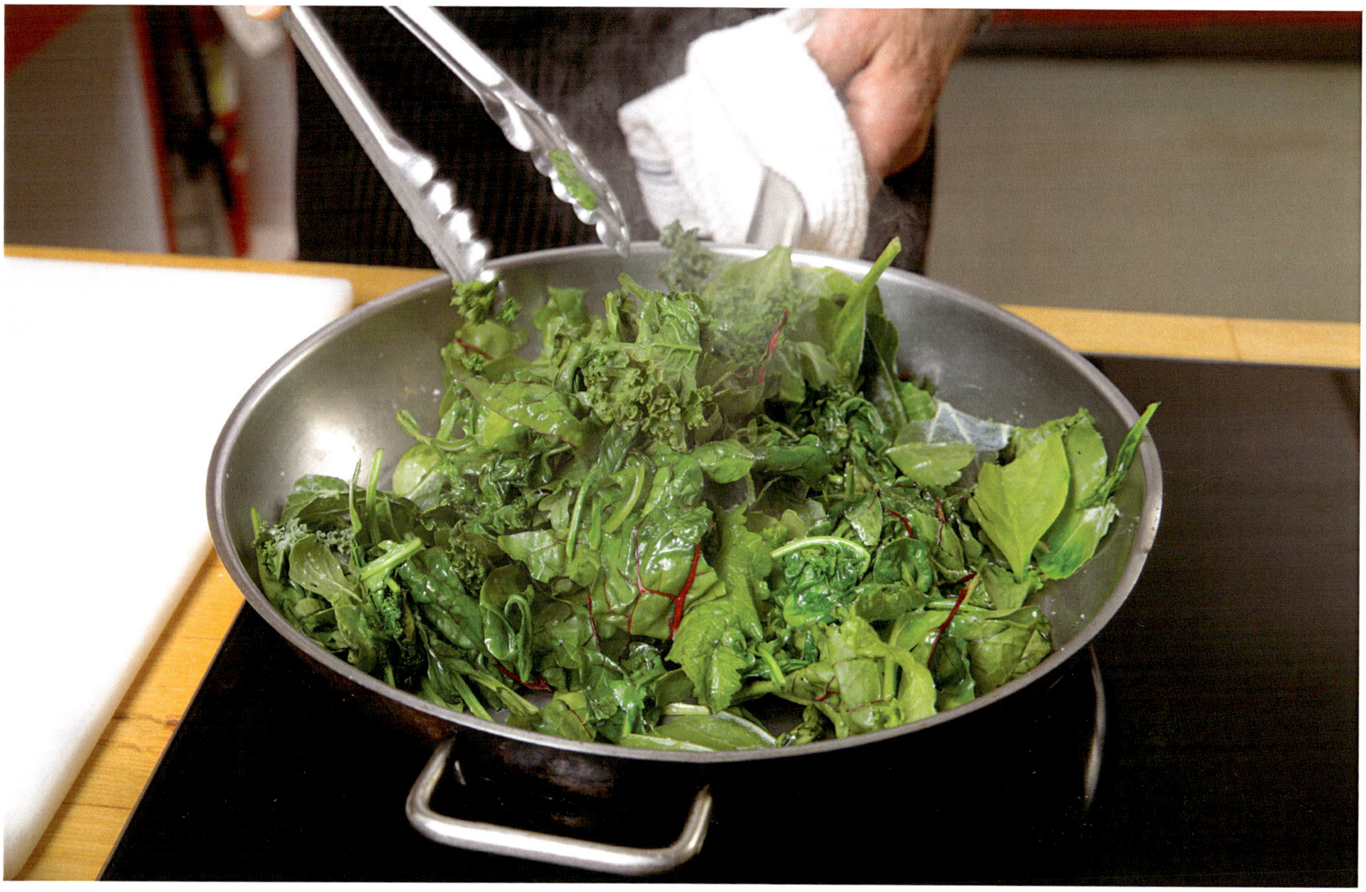

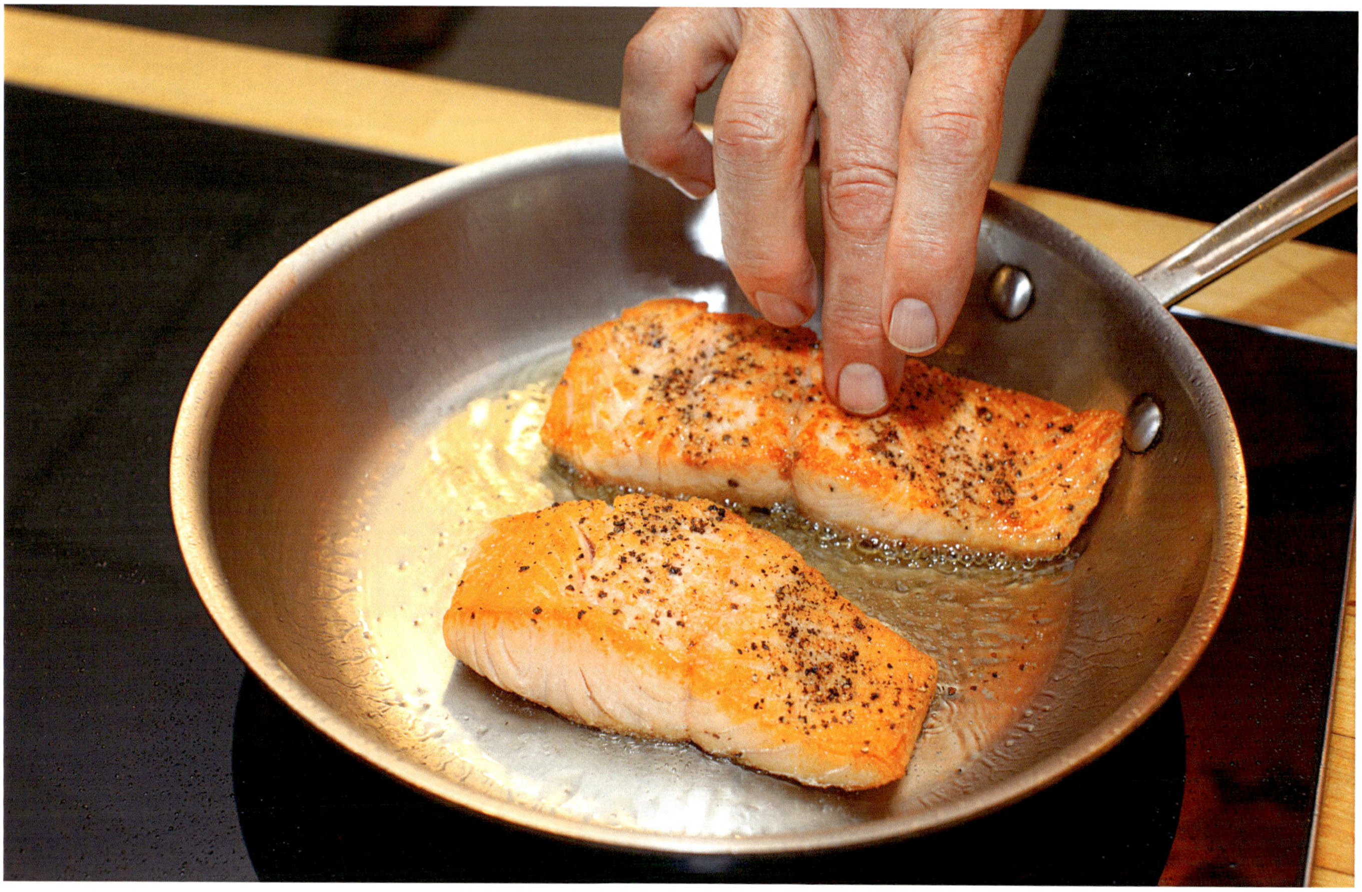

EMULSIFICATION TECHNIQUES

It sounds scientific but emulsification is a basic part of cooking. It's about blending oil and vinegar together without having it separate, and the technique is to whip fast and to slowly add the oil. The vinegar or citrus juice, the emulsifier and any seasonings you like are placed in a mixing bowl or blender and while whipping, the oil is slowly added. The goal is to create a smooth and evenly flavored sauce, and is mainly reserved for salad dressings, vinaigrettes and mayonnaise, although it has other applications in more advanced cookery.

Emulsifiers include, but are not limited to, mustards, egg yolks, fruit purées, vegetable purées, peanut butter and tomato paste. The emulsifier is also an integral flavor component of the sauce.

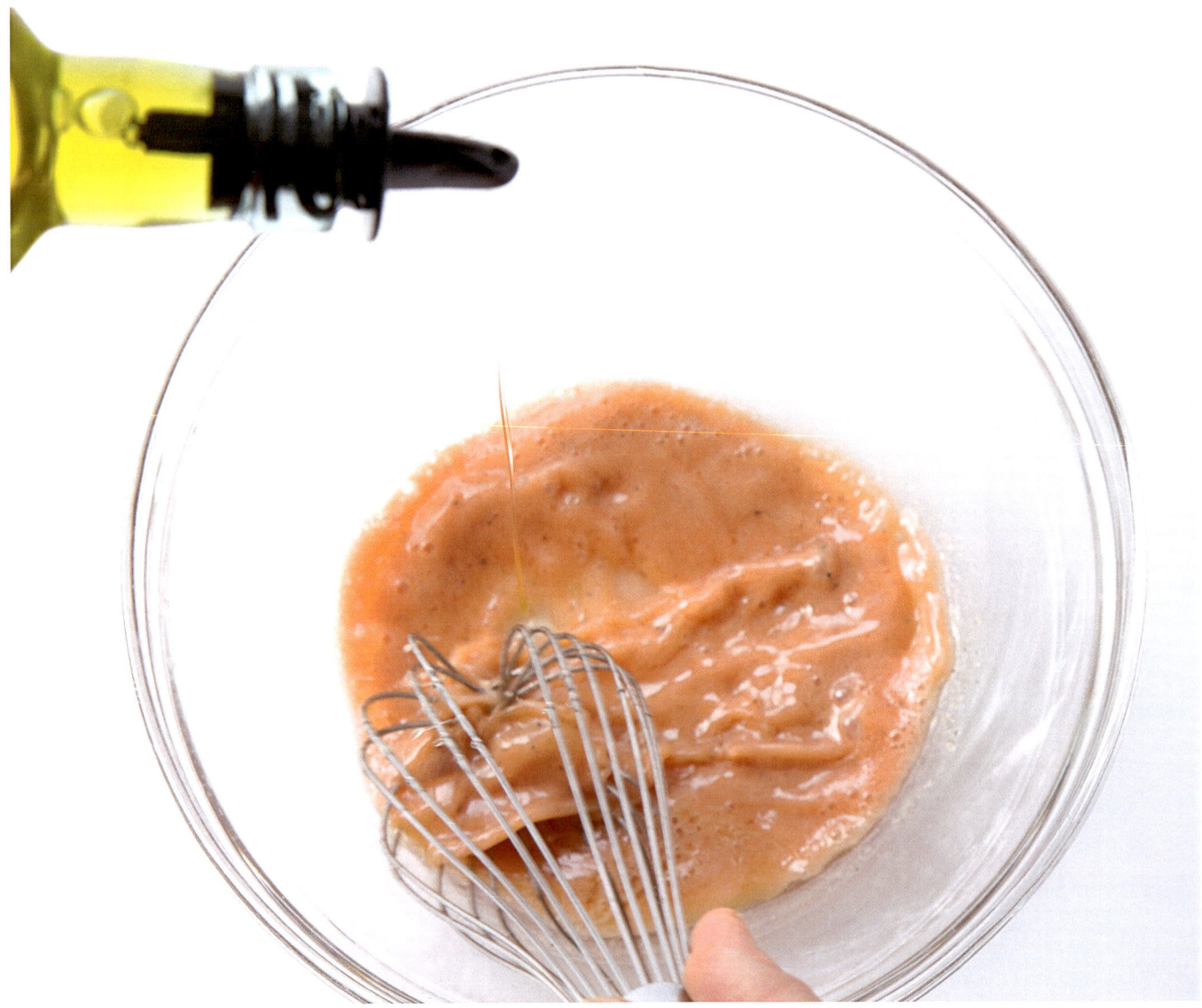

SEASONING TECHNIQUES

Everyone's palate is different. While we know that the main five flavors that we taste are sweet, sour, bitter, salty and umami or earthiness, every palate picks these up somewhat differently. In other words, our taste buds are as unique as we are.

The main ingredients we season with are salt, pepper, spices and acidity. Under these fall items like soy sauce, curry, hot sauce, lemon juice, and vinegar to name a paltry few. A common example of this is the Caesar salad. The saltiness comes from the anchovies, the acidity comes from lemon juice, and the pepper comes from Tabasco.

All of these flavors should be "TO TASTE". My best advice is to put in a small amount and then taste and adjust the seasonings as necessary. A good starting point, if needed, is ½ teaspoon salt, ¼ teaspoon ground black pepper, 1 tablespoon vinegar or lemon juice, and a dash of hot sauce.

If necessary, adjust the flavors by adding a little more of what you think it needs: sometimes it's just a pinch of salt. If it's still not quite right, take a sip of water and rinse your palate. This will reset your taste buds.

Over-seasoning happens to the best of us. Your meal may be less enjoyable but it won't be ruined. Practice won't make perfect but it will make precision.

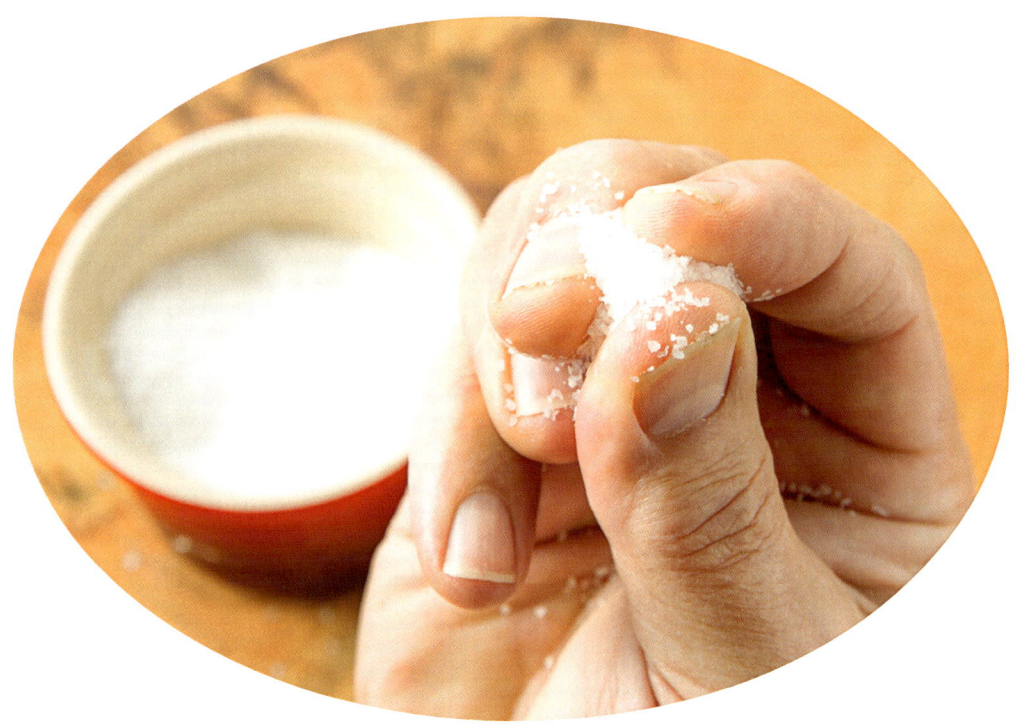

CHECKING FOR DONENESS IN PROTEINS

I use a digital meat thermometer for thicker meats that are an inch and a half thick or more. For thinner cuts I use the "touch technique". Make the okay sign with one hand. Tap, don't press the fingers together. With the index finger of your other hand, press the muscle on the palm of your hand just below the thumb. This is what rare feels like. Next, make the okay sign using your middle finger and press the same muscle. This is medium rare. Making the okay sign with your ring finger and touching same muscle is medium. Okay sign with baby finger, touching same muscle is medium-well.

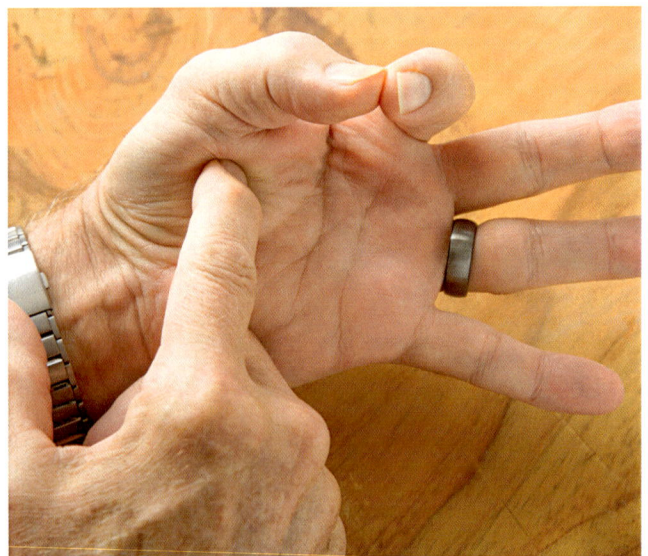
Rare

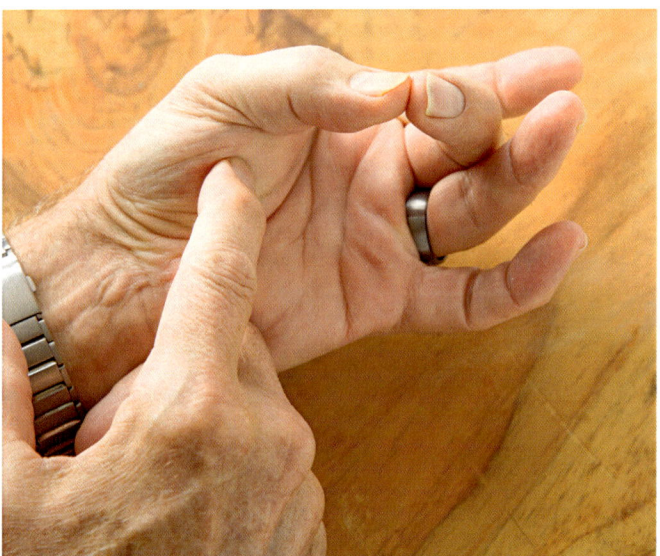
Medium Rare

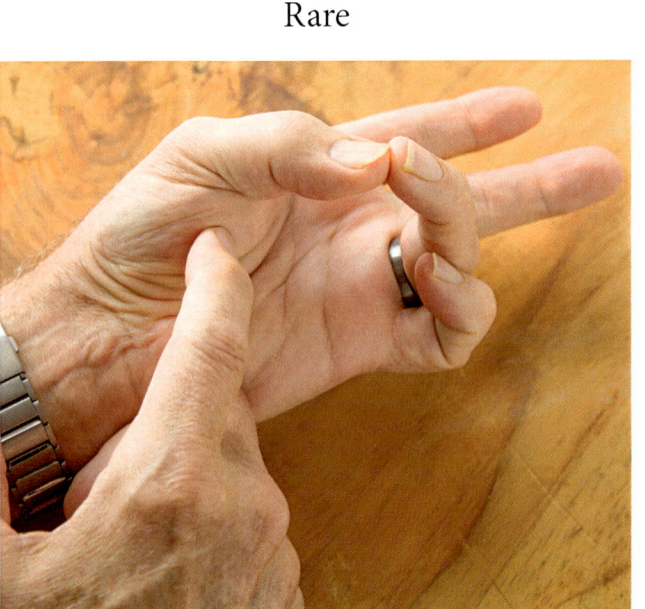
Medium

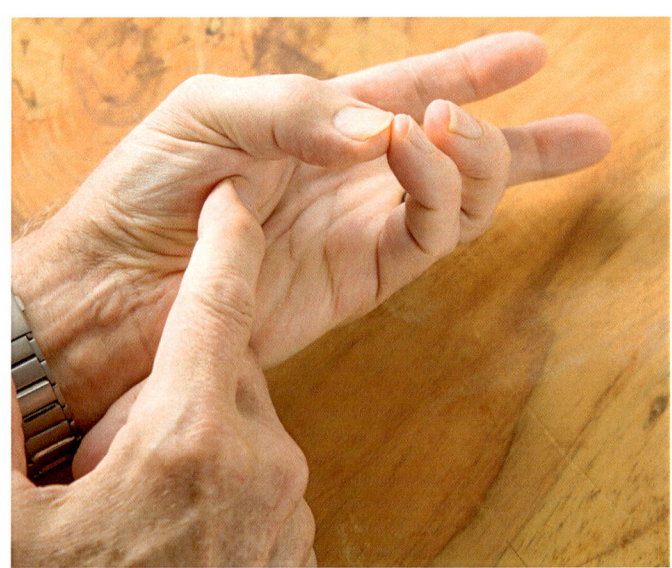
Medium Well

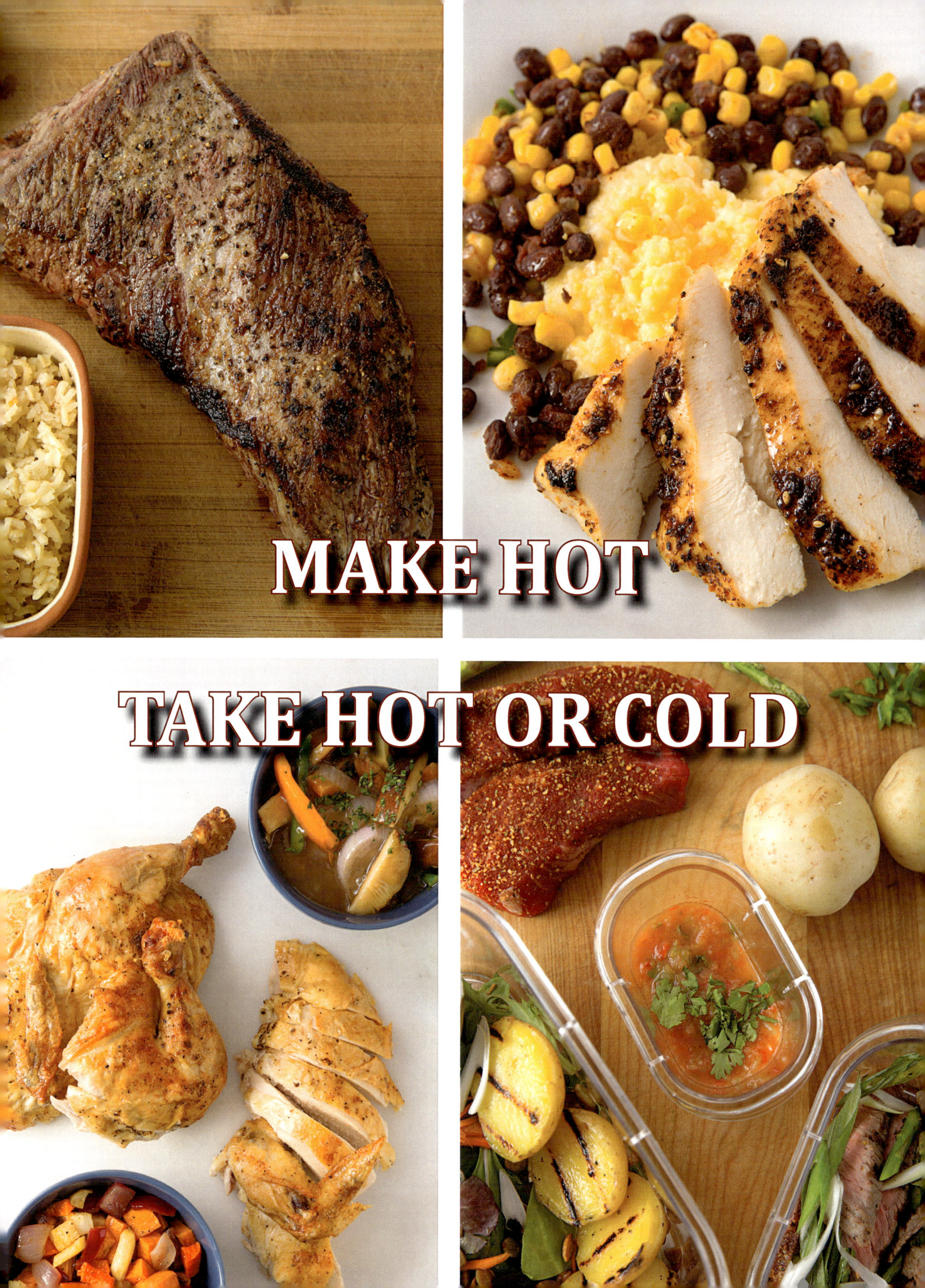

MAKE HOT

TAKE HOT OR COLD

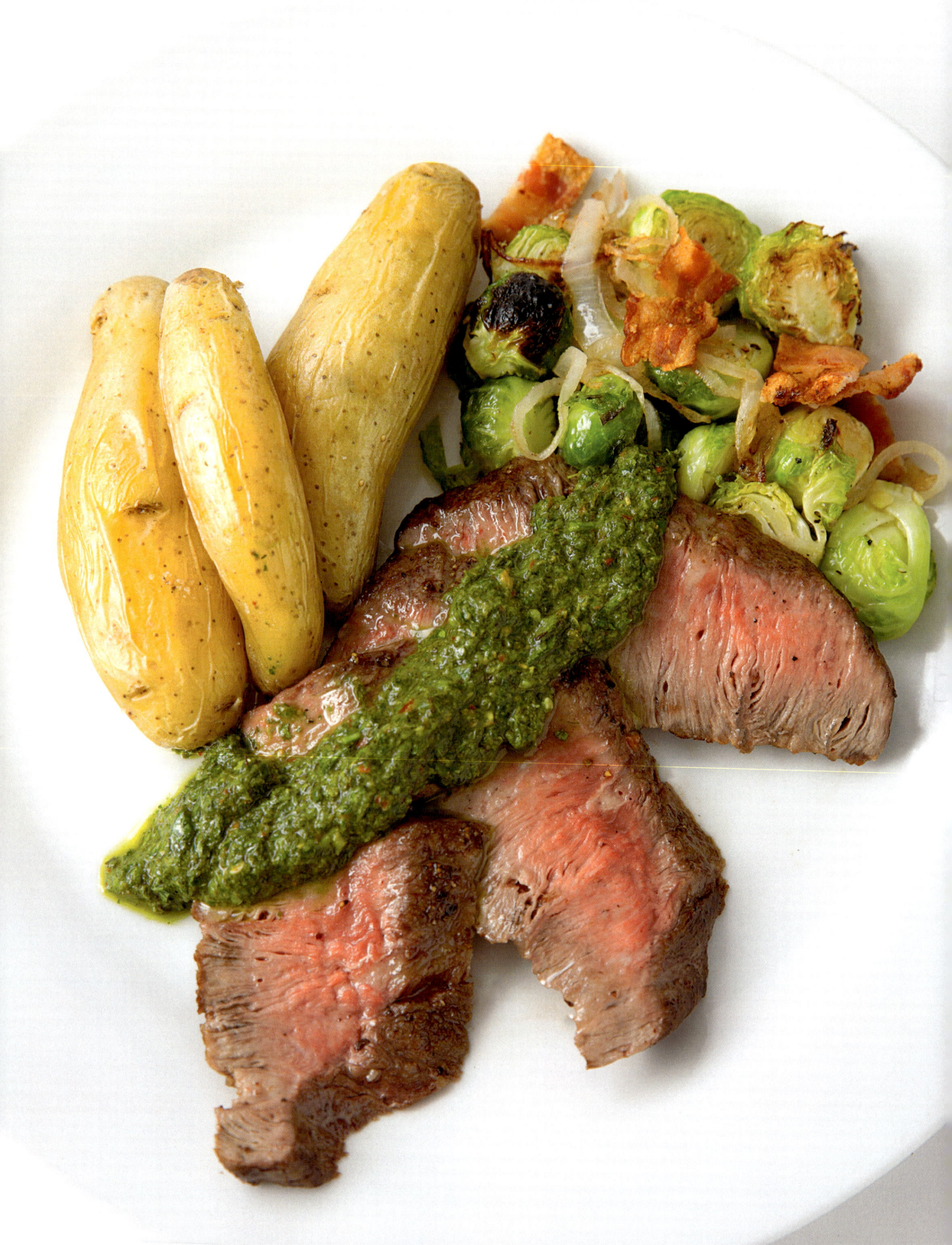

PAN-SEARED FLATIRON STEAKS

So-called because it resembles an old-fashioned flatiron, this cut of meat comes from the shoulder of the cow, and offers a good value and tender steak that can be pan-seared to perfection. As with all cuts of meat, resting before slicing is essential with a flatiron steak. The highly-flavored Argentinean-inspired sauce, full of herbs, garlic and vinegar is a natural accompaniment, and if you haven't ever paired them before, Brussels sprouts and bacon are a match made in heaven!

Make Hot and Fresh
Chimichurri Sauce, Bacon Roasted Brussels Sprouts, Roasted Fingerling Potatoes
Makes 4 Servings

Serve The Next Day Cold
Cherry Tomatoes, Cucumber, Balsamic Vinaigrette
Makes 1 Serving

Roasted Fingerling Potatoes

2 lbs fingerling potatoes, washed and cut into 1-inch pieces
Salt and pepper
2 Tbsp olive oil

Preheat oven to 375°F.

Place the potatoes in a large pot and cover with cold water. Add large pinch of salt and bring to a boil. Cook the potatoes for 5 minutes, then drain and allow to air dry.

Mix the potatoes with the oil, salt and pepper in a medium mixing bowl and toss to coat. Spread the potatoes evenly on a metal sheet pan and place in the oven. Cook until the potatoes are softened and lightly browned, approximately 25-30 minutes. Remove from oven and serve immediately, or cover and keep warm.

Bacon Roasted Brussels Sprouts

1 lb Brussels sprouts
6 oz bacon, chopped
2 Tbsp olive oil
2 shallots, thinly sliced
Salt and pepper

Preheat oven to 350°F.

Trim the stem ends of the Brussels sprouts and remove any yellow outer leaves. Cut into quarters.

Heat a large skillet over medium-high heat. Add the bacon and cook until crisp, about 4 minutes. Remove the bacon to paper towels and drain well. Set aside.

Pour off excess bacon grease, then add the oil and the shallots to the skillet and cook briefly, about 20 seconds. Add the Brussels sprouts to the pan, season with salt and pepper, and toss to coat with the oil. Sauté briefly, top with the bacon and place in the oven. Cook for about 12-15 minutes, or until tender-crisp. Serve immediately or keep warm until ready to serve.

Chimichurri Sauce

4 cloves garlic
½ cup olive oil
¼ cup red wine vinegar
Juice of half a lemon
2 tsp dried oregano
½ cup dried parsley
½ tsp crushed red
   pepper
Salt and pepper

Combine all ingredients in a medium bowl and blend using a hand blender (or combine in a blender) just until slightly chunky or has reached the desired consistency. Taste for seasoning and adjust as needed. Will keep, covered and refrigerated for up to 5 days. Makes about 1 cup

Pan-Seared Flatiron Steaks

20-24 oz flatiron steak
Salt and pepper
Olive oil

Dry the steak with paper towels. Season both sides of the steak with salt and pepper.

Heat a large skillet on high heat. When hot, add the olive oil, then add the steak. Reduce heat to medium and cook for 6-8 minutes on each side, until the steak is brown on each side and just firm to the touch. The internal temperature should be 120-125°F. Remove and let rest for about 3-5 minutes, then slice very thin and serve. Serve immediately.

SERVE THE NEXT DAY COLD
Cherry Tomatoes, Cucumber, Balsamic Vinaigrette

Balsamic Vinaigrette

¼ cup balsamic vinegar
1 Tbsp Dijon mustard
1 small shallot, minced
1 clove garlic, minced
Salt and pepper
½ cup extra-virgin olive oil

Optional, 1-2 Tbsp stemmed and minced fresh herbs (e.g. basil, oregano, tarragon, Italian parsley, thyme, chives)

In a medium mixing bowl or food processor, whisk together the balsamic vinegar, mustard, shallot, garlic, salt and pepper. While whisking, slowly drizzle in the olive oil. Taste and adjust the seasonings and add the fresh herbs, if desired. Cover and refrigerate until ready to serve. Will keep covered and refrigerated for up to 3 days. Makes about ¾ cup

To Assemble

About 4-6 cherry tomatoes

¼ cucumber, sliced thin

⅓ cup Bacon Roasted Brussels Sprouts

½ cup sliced Roasted Fingerling Potatoes

5-6 oz thinly sliced Pan-Seared Flatiron Steaks

Large handful mixed greens

¼ cup Balsamic Vinaigrette

¼ cup pistachios, roasted, salted and crushed

Pack the raw vegetables in one travel container, the sprouts, potatoes and steak in a second container, the vinaigrette in a third, and the nuts in a fourth. When ready to serve, place all ingredients in a serving bowl and toss together.

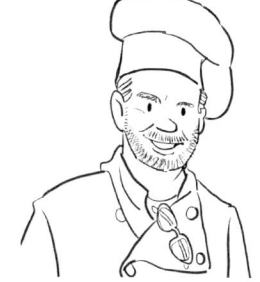

As with all cuts of meat, it is essential to rest flatiron steak before slicing — this means that the meat will lose less juice when it is carved and ensures a tastier, juicier steak.

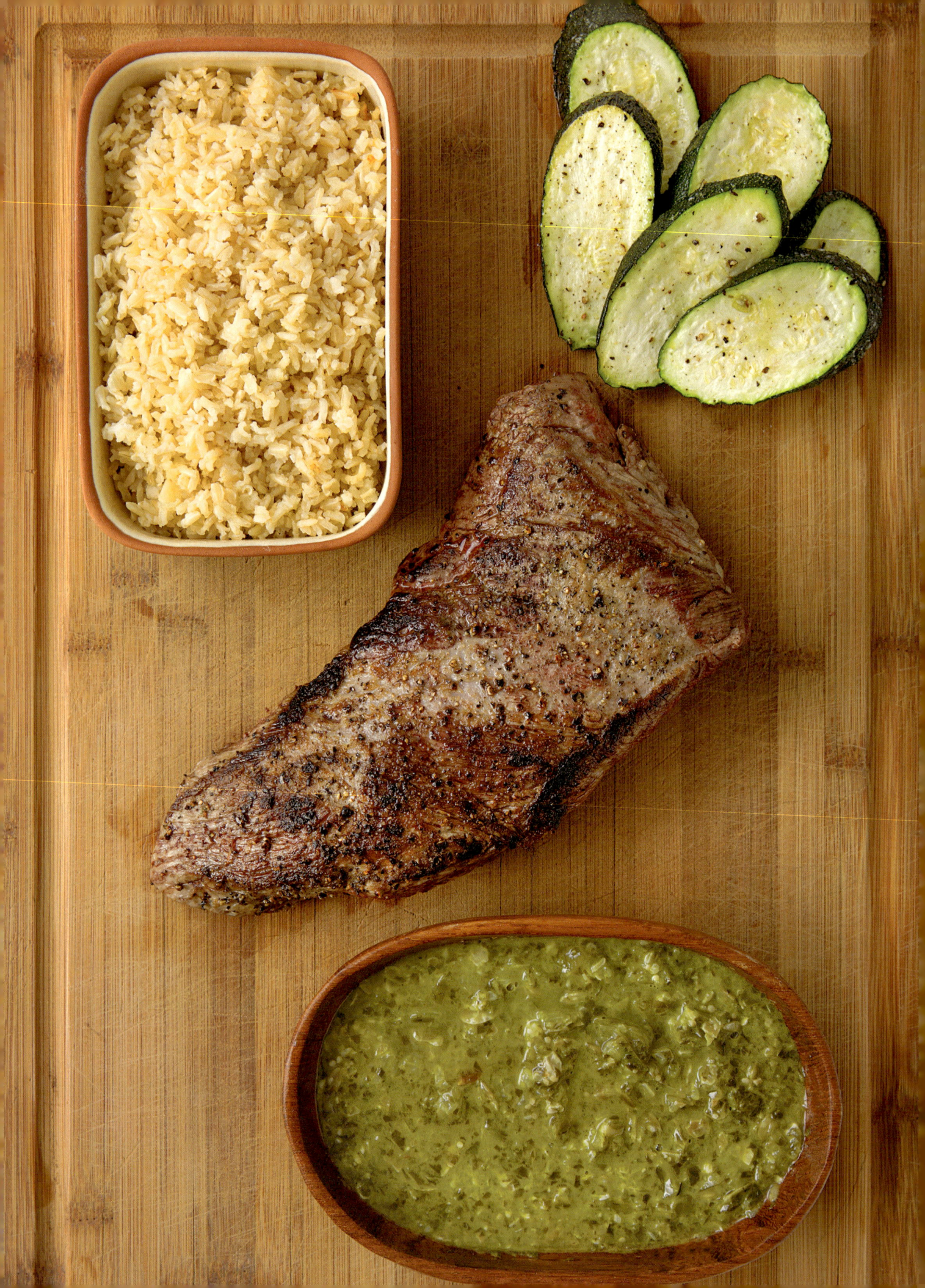

TRIANGLE TIP ROAST

Roasting is my favorite way to cook many vegetables, as they retain their texture and it helps to bring out their flavor. Always make sure you lay out the vegetables flat on a baking tray, so they cook evenly, and never stack them. Roasted vegetables also reheat magnificently. Brown rice is a delicious whole grain, but needs to be treated differently from white rice and requires a longer cooking time. This mole recipe is courtesy of my good friend, Cathy Harakopis, who learnt it while traveling around Central America. None of the mole ingredients need precise measurement.

Make Hot and Fresh
Tomatillo Mole, Roasted Zucchini, Brown Rice
Makes 4 Servings

Serve The Next Day Cold
Bed of Mixed Greens
Makes 1 Serving

Brown Rice

1 cup long grain brown rice

3 cups chicken stock
Salt and pepper

Place all ingredients in a medium saucepot. Stir once and bring to a boil. Reduce to a simmer and cover. Cook for 40-45 minutes or until rice is tender and all liquid is absorbed.

Keep covered until ready to serve or uncover, let cool, and reheat when ready to eat. Rice may also be served cold. Makes about 2½ cups

Tomatillo Mole

⅓ cup raw pumpkin seeds

4 oz tomatillos, hulled and washed

½ cup chopped arugula
¼ cup chopped yellow onion

¼ cup chopped spinach
2 Tbsp chopped cilantro
1 jalapeño, seeded and de-ribbed

1 clove garlic
Salt
1-2 cups chicken stock
2 Tbsp olive oil

Heat a medium skillet on medium heat. When hot, add the pumpkin seeds and lightly toast for 1-2 minutes until starting to puff. Transfer to a blender and add the tomatillos, arugula, onion, spinach, cilantro, jalapeño, garlic and salt. Add 1 cup of stock and purée until smooth.

Heat a large pot on medium heat and add the oil. Add the mix carefully, as it will sizzle as it hits the hot oil. Add a little more stock to the blender to swish out all the remaining mixture and add to the pot. Simmer until the mole just starts to thicken. If it separates and looks like scrambled eggs, just add a little more stock.

Remove, taste and adjust the seasonings and let cool. Makes about 2 cups

Roasted Zucchini

2 zucchinis
1 Tbsp olive oil, or to
   coat
Salt and pepper

Preheat oven to 350°F.

Trim the zucchini and cut on a 45° bias, about ½-inch thick. Lay out on a sheet pan, without stacking, and brush with the olive oil. Sprinkle with the salt and pepper. Place in the oven and roast for 8-10 minutes, or until the zucchini is bendable to the touch and tender to the bite. Remove and serve, or let cool.

Triangle Tip Roast

1½-2 lbs triangle tip
   roast
Salt and pepper
2 Tbsp salad oil

Preheat oven to 375°F.

Heat a large skillet on high heat. Dry the meat on paper towels. Season both sides of the roast with salt and pepper.

When the skillet is hot, add the oil and lay in the roast. Brown lightly for about 2 minutes on each side. Place in the oven and reduce the heat to 350°F. Roast for 20-25 minutes, depending on the thickness of the roast, or until it reaches an internal temperature of 125°F for medium-rare, or to desired degree of doneness.

When done, remove from the oven and let rest for 5 minutes. Slice thin and serve.

SERVE THE NEXT DAY COLD
Bed of Mixed Greens

To Assemble

Large handful mixed
   greens
5-6 spears Roasted
   Zucchini
5-6 oz sliced Roasted
   Triangle Tip Roast
½ cup Brown Rice
¼ cup Tomatillo Mole
Any other raw, sliced
   or shaved vegetables
   (e.g. carrots, snap peas,
   mushrooms, celery,
   green onions, fennel,
   bell peppers)

Pack all ingredients in separate travel containers. When ready to serve, place all ingredients in a serving bowl and toss together.

DRY RUB GRILLED TRIANGLE TIP STEAK

Triangle Tip is my favorite cut of beef. It is well-priced and extremely versatile, which is why it is the single most important cut of meat for me in both teaching and catering. Plus it's delicious, and stays tender when cold, so is an excellent choice for make-and-take meals. The Dry Rub can go with any meat to offer a Central American flavor, so it may be one place where you want to measure the salt and pepper. And these are my wife's favorite potatoes!

Make Hot and Fresh
Roasted Tomato Salsa, Grilled New Potatoes, Roasted Asparagus
Makes 4 Servings

Serve The Next Day Cold
Bed of Mixed Greens, Scallions, Roasted Pumpkin Seeds
Makes 1 Serving

Grilled New Potatoes

1 lb new potatoes, any color

Salt and pepper
2-3 Tbsp olive oil

Preheat grill or indoor grill plate.

Wash potatoes and place in a medium saucepot. Cover with water, add a pinch of salt and place on stove. Bring to a boil, reduce to a simmer and cook for 15-20 minutes or until potatoes are tender. Drain and let cool.

Cut potatoes in half and place in a medium mixing bowl. Add salt, pepper and olive oil and toss to coat. Place on the grill, cut side down and cook 3-5 minutes, or until potatoes have nice grill marks. Remove and serve when ready. Potatoes may be served hot or cold.

Roasted Tomato Salsa

3 small tomatoes
1 Anaheim chili, stemmed, split and seeded

1 small yellow onion, sliced ¼-inch thick
1 Tbsp olive oil
Salt and pepper
2 cloves garlic, peeled and crushed

1-2 limes, juiced
Optional, 2 Tbsp stemmed and chopped cilantro

Preheat oven to 350°F.

Core, split and squeeze the seeds and juice out of the tomatoes. Place the chili, sliced onion and tomatoes on a baking tray. Lightly coat with olive oil and sprinkle with salt and pepper. Place in the oven and roast for about 20 minutes, until the vegetables are soft. Remove and let cool.

Place the chili, onion, tomatoes and garlic in a food processor and blend well. Add half the lime juice, then season with salt and pepper to taste. Add more lime juice as needed.

Transfer to a serving bowl and stir in the cilantro, if using. Will keep covered and refrigerated for up to 3 days. Makes about 2 cups

Roasted Asparagus

1 bundle asparagus,
   woody ends cut off
1 Tbsp olive oil or to coat
Salt and pepper

Preheat oven to 350°F.

Lay the asparagus out on a metal sheet pan without stacking. Brush with the olive oil and sprinkle with salt and pepper. Place in the oven and roast for about 7-12 minutes, depending on the thickness of the spears, or until the spears are bendable and tender to the bite. Remove and serve, or let cool.

Dry Rub Grilled Triangle Tip Steaks

2 Tbsp Ancho chili
   powder
1 tsp salt
1 tsp black pepper
2 tsp sugar
2 tsp dried oregano
4 each 5-6 oz triangle tip
   steaks, about 1-inch
   thick
2-4 Tbsp olive oil

In a mixing bowl, combine the chili powder, salt, pepper, sugar and oregano. Liberally coat the steaks with the dry mix. Cover and refrigerate for at least 30 minutes or overnight. Brush the steaks with the olive oil when ready to cook.

Heat a grill or cast iron skillet on high heat.

When hot, place the steaks on the grill or skillet. Cook for 5-6 minutes, then turn over and cook for an additional 5-6 minutes. At this point, the steaks are medium rare. Add 1-2 more minutes per degree of desired doneness. Remove and set aside to cool slightly.

Indoor grill plates can play a big role in your everyday cooking. They will work on top of your stove (or on top of your outdoor grill) so you don't need to fire up the barbecue every time you want a little grill flavor. And nothing falls through the grates!

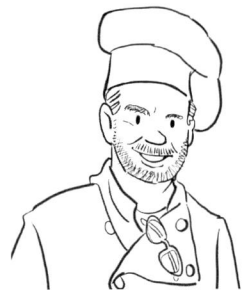

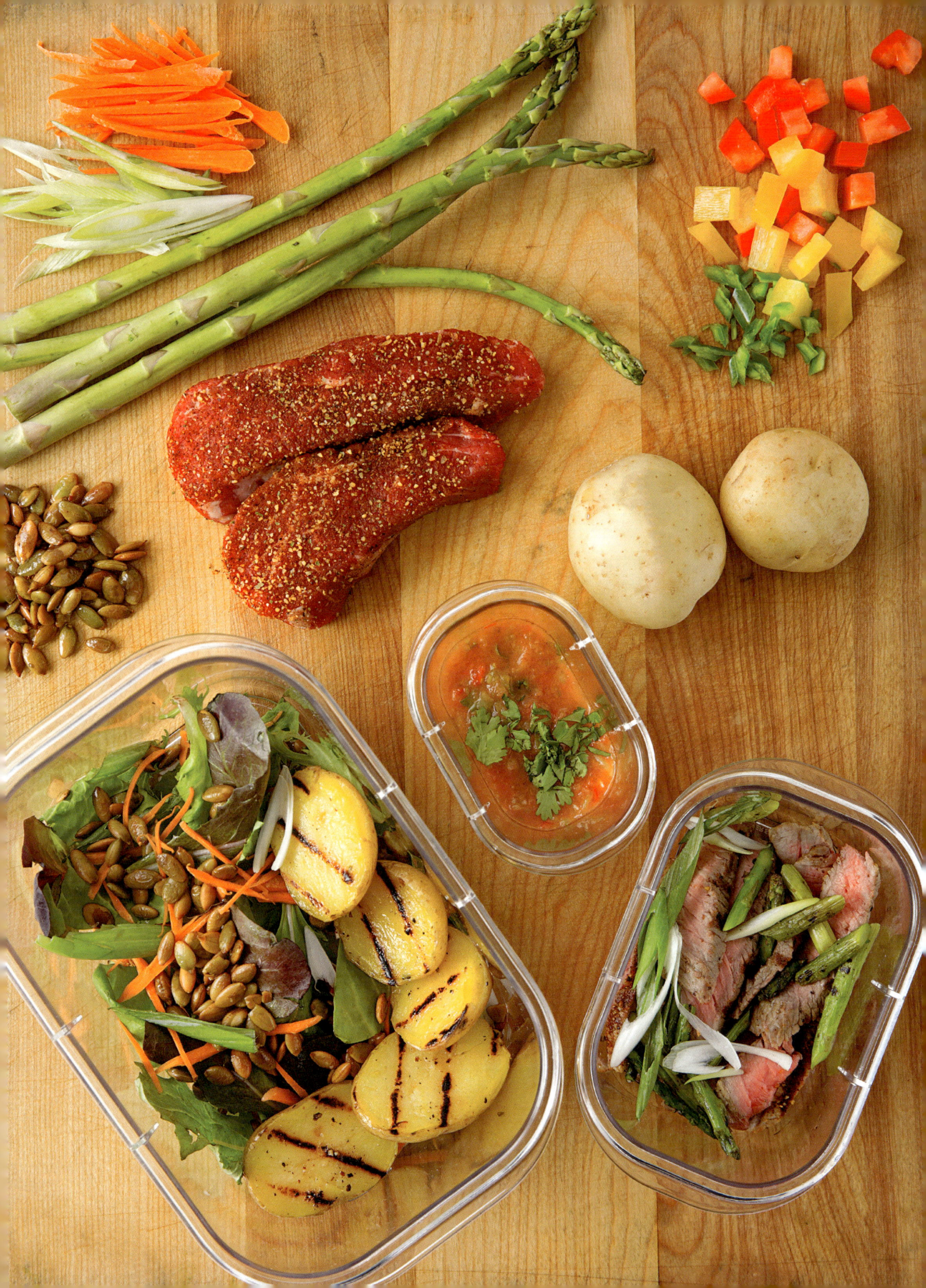

SERVE THE NEXT DAY COLD
Bed of Mixed Greens, Scallions, Roasted Pumpkin Seeds

Large handful mixed greens

¼ cup chopped scallions

1 Tbsp roasted and salted pumpkin seeds

½ cup Grilled New Potatoes

1 Dry Rub Grilled Triangle Tip Steak, sliced thin

⅓ cup Roasted Tomato Salsa

Any other raw, sliced or shaved vegetables (e.g. carrots, snap peas, mushrooms, celery, green onions, fennel, bell peppers)

To Assemble

Pack all ingredients in separate containers. When ready to serve, place all ingredients in a serving bowl and toss together.

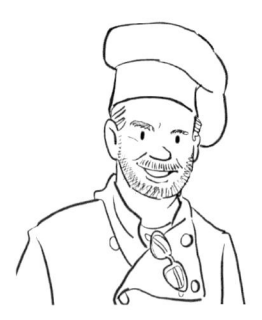

I often have a jar of roasted tomatoes, which I cover with olive oil, in my fridge. Apart from having so many uses in cooking, they can also be used as a snack, appetizer or part of an upscale charcuterie or antipasto plate.

GRILLED FLATIRON STEAK

I always try to use everyday vegetables in my cooking. Exotic varieties certainly have their place, but running around all over town for that elusive ingredient really cuts into your cooking (and eating) time. I prefer to stick to the humble vegetables that I know and love, and experiment with varied cooking methods and different seasonings to really elevate their flavor profile and expand their versatility – hence the cauliflower risotto I have included here. Fortunately, most markets now carry a nice variety of mushrooms, all of which can work in the Wild Mushroom Salsa.

Make Hot and Fresh
Wild Mushroom Salsa, Cauliflower Risotto,
Sautéed New Potatoes
Makes 4 Servings

Serve The Next Day Hot
Makes 1 Serving

Wild Mushroom Salsa

⅓ cup olive oil
3 Tbsp balsamic vinegar
3-4 cloves garlic, minced
1½ Tbsp fajita seasoning mix
Salt and pepper
Scant 1 Tbsp stemmed and minced fresh thyme
1 lb assorted wild mushrooms, cleaned and stemmed
¼ cup stemmed and thinly sliced arugula
Large pinch dried crushed red pepper

In a large mixing bowl, combine the olive oil, balsamic vinegar, garlic, fajita seasoning, salt, pepper, and thyme. Add the wild mushrooms and gently toss to coat. Set aside to marinate for 15 minutes or up to 2 hours.

Heat an indoor grill plate on medium heat. Remove the mushrooms from the marinade and gently scrape off any excess. Set the remaining marinade aside. When the grill is hot, place the mushrooms on the cook surface and grill until they are tender, turning once, for about 3-5 minutes. Remove and let cool.

Coarsely chop the mushrooms and gently toss with the arugula, red pepper and remaining marinade. Taste to adjust seasonings. Cover and refrigerate. Bring to room temperature before serving. Makes about 2½ cups

Cauliflower Risotto

½ head cauliflower
2 Tbsp olive oil
1 small onion, diced
2 cloves garlic, chopped
Salt and pepper
¾ cup chicken stock (plus more as necessary)

Break the cauliflower into florets and place in a food processor. Pulse chop until the cauliflower resembles rice.

Heat a large, high-sided skillet over medium heat. When hot, add the oil, then add the onion, and sauté for about 3-4 minutes, or until translucent. Add the cauliflower and the garlic, season with salt and pepper, and sauté for 1-2 more minutes.

Add the chicken stock and bring to a simmer. Cover and cook for about 6-8 minutes, or until the cauliflower is tender. Keep warm until ready to serve. Makes about 3 cups

Sautéed New Potatoes

1½ lbs red new potatoes,
  washed
Pinch salt
2 Tbsp olive oil
1 Tbsp stemmed and
  chopped Italian parsley
2 cloves garlic, minced
Ground black pepper
½ Tbsp paprika

Cut the potatoes in half and slice in ¼-inch slices. Place in a medium pot, cover with cold water and add a large pinch of salt. Put on high heat and bring to a boil. Reduce the temperature to a simmer and cook for about 3 minutes. Remove, drain and let dry.

Heat a large skillet on high heat. When hot, add the oil and potatoes. Reduce heat to medium and cook until the potatoes are lightly browned. Stir and continue to cook for about 10-12 minutes, stirring occasionally, until the potatoes are tender to the bite. Remove and toss with the parsley, garlic, pepper and paprika.

Keep warm until ready to serve.

Grilled Flatiron Steak

20-24 oz flatiron steak
Salt and pepper
Olive oil

Heat a grill on medium-high heat.

Dry the steak with paper towels. Trim away any firm white tissue or gristle. Season both sides of the steak with salt and pepper, and brush with olive oil. Place the steak on the grill. Cook for 6-8 minutes on each side, until the steak is brown on each side and just firm to the touch. The internal temperature should be 120-125°F. Remove and let rest for about 3 minutes, then slice very thin and serve. Serve immediately.

SERVE THE NEXT DAY HOT

½ cup Sautéed New
  Potatoes
4-5 oz Grilled Flatiron
  Steak
½ cup Cauliflower
  Risotto
½ cup Wild Mushroom
  Salsa

Place potatoes in a microwave-proof plastic container, topped with steak, risotto, and salsa. When ready to eat, sprinkle 1 Tbsp water on top and loosely cover with the lid, then reheat for 3-4 minutes or until hot all the way through.

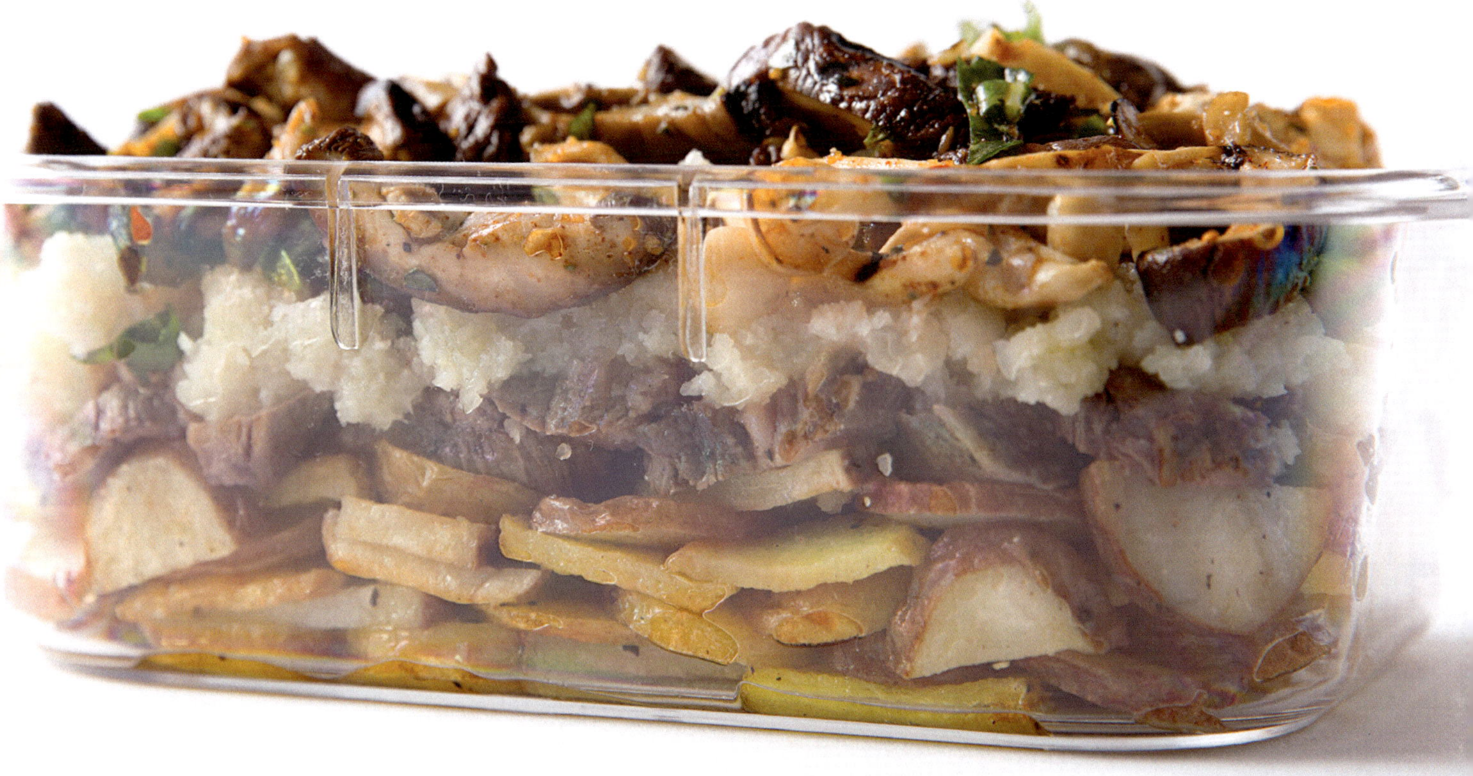

Don't limit yourself to the humble button mushroom — supermarkets and grocery stores now offer a fantastic range of wild mushrooms in their produce departments. From earthy Shiitakes and meaty Morels, to more delicate Chanterelles, make a point of trying something new and experimenting with all the different varieties out there. You can also rehydrate dried mushrooms for a very intense and more concentrated flavor.

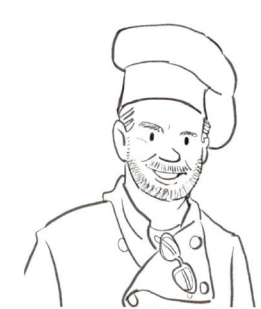

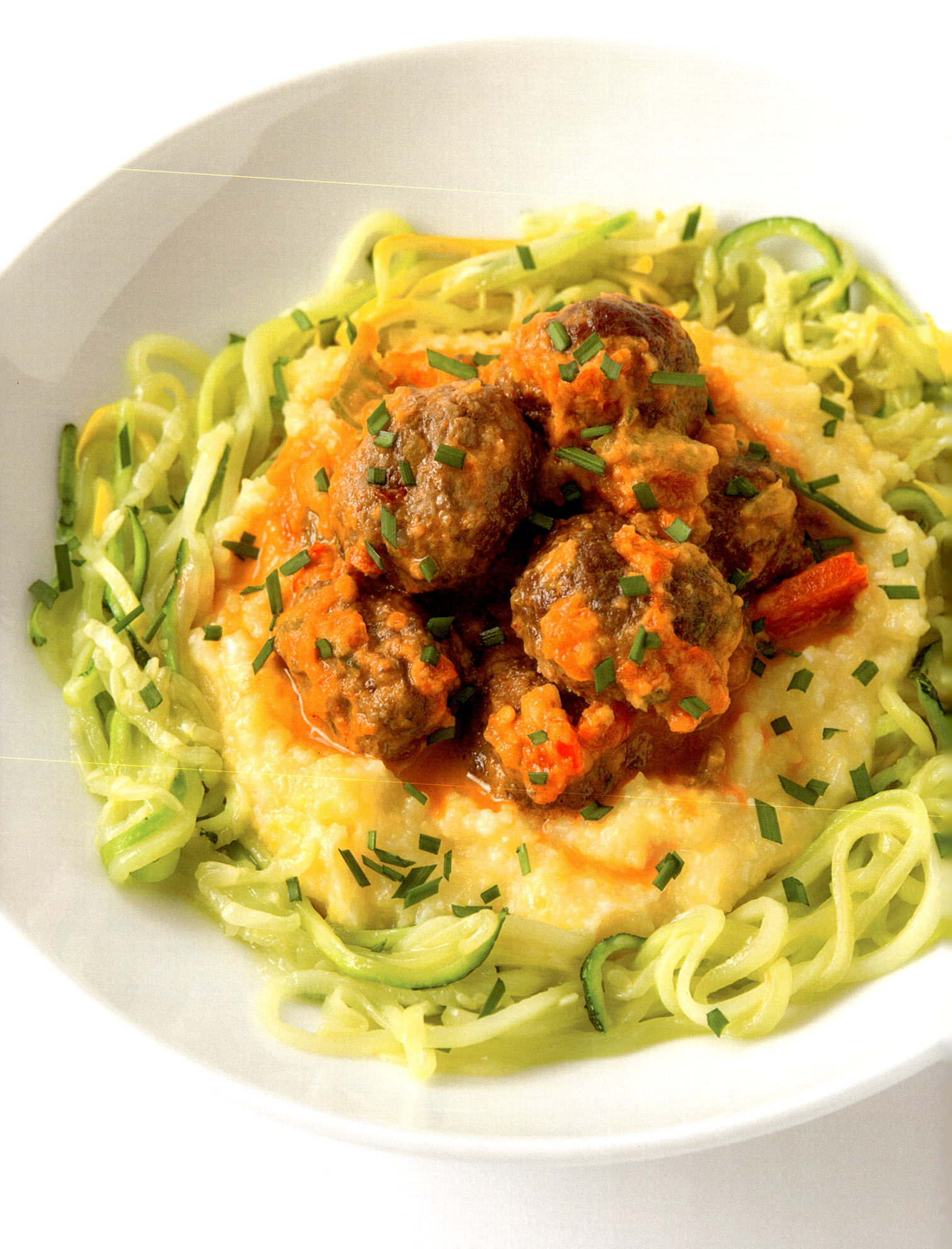

SPICY BISON MEATBALLS

The components in this recipe define this cookbook. They are versatile; they are healthy; they are delicious. In this recipe, I have used ground bison, which should be readily available in your local supermarket or grocery store. Bison has a lot of health advantages over other proteins which is why I'm using it here, but you can use any ground protein in its place. The Tomato Pepper Piperade is an amazing healthy upgrade from your everyday marinara sauce and also goes well with beef, chicken, pork, turkey, etc. The Squash Noodles make a fun, tasty pasta-like accompaniment to many dishes without the refined flour found in regular pastas.

Make Hot and Fresh
Tomato Pepper Piperade, Squash Noodles
Makes 6 Servings

Serve The Next Day Hot
Makes 1 Serving

Tomato Pepper Piperade

2 green bell peppers, stemmed and seeded

2 red bell peppers, stemmed and seeded

4 medium tomatoes, cored and cut in half

4-6 Tbsp olive oil

4 cloves garlic, minced

1 tsp crushed red pepper flakes

4 Tbsp stemmed and minced oregano

2-4 Tbsp white wine vinegar

Salt and pepper

Preheat broiler.

Lay the peppers flat on a metal sheet pan skin side up and brush lightly with some of the olive oil. Place the tomatoes on the sheet pan and lightly coat with olive oil. Place the pan under the broiler and cook until the skins blacken on the tomatoes and peppers, 3-4 minutes. Remove and let cool. When cool enough to handle, remove the blackened skin from the peppers and tomatoes. Julienne the peppers and roughly chop the tomatoes.

Heat a large skillet over medium heat. When hot, add 2 Tbsp olive oil and the garlic and cook for approximately 20-30 seconds, being careful not to burn the garlic. Add the peppers, tomatoes, red pepper flakes and oregano, stirring lightly. Cook for 3-4 minutes until heated through, then season with the vinegar, salt and pepper. Transfer to a blender and purée. Return the sauce to the pot and taste and adjust the seasonings. Makes about 2 cups

Squash Noodles

1 zucchini
1 yellow squash
2 Tbsp olive oil
Salt and pepper

Trim the ends off of the squash and cut in 3- to 4-inch lengths. Using a spiralizer, cut the squash into noodle shaped threads.

Heat a medium skillet on medium heat. When hot, add the oil and the squash. Season with salt and pepper and cook for about 2-3 minutes, stirring occasionally, until the squash is tender to the bite. Keep warm until ready to serve.

Spicy Bison Meatballs

2 lbs ground bison
1-2 canned chipotle
    peppers, minced

1 tsp smoked paprika
1 tsp onion powder
Salt and pepper

Preheat oven to 350°F.

Combine the meat, peppers and spices in a bowl. Form into 24 balls, about 1⅓ oz each. These can be made ahead, if kept covered and refrigerated.

When ready to cook, put the meatballs on a sheet pan and place in the oven. Cook the meatballs for about 12-14 minutes, or until the meat is springy to the touch. Remove and keep warm until ready to serve.

To Assemble

Optional, 2 Tbsp grated
Parmesan cheese

Toss together the meatballs, piperade and squash noodles and serve with grated Parmesan cheese, if desired.

SERVE THE NEXT DAY HOT

½ cup Squash Noodles
4-5 oz Spicy Bison
    Meatballs
½ cup Tomato Pepper
    Piperade

Place squash noodles in a microwave-proof plastic container, then top with meatballs and cover with piperade. When ready to eat, sprinkle with 1 Tbsp water, loosely place the lid on top and reheat for 3-4 minutes or until hot all the way through.

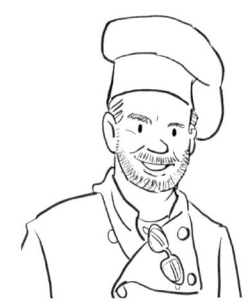

Spiralizers are all the rage nowadays, as people embrace more plant-based diets, and a side of squash "noodles" creates a fresh, nutritious and colorful addition to your meal. A sturdy spiralizer can even cut root vegetables.

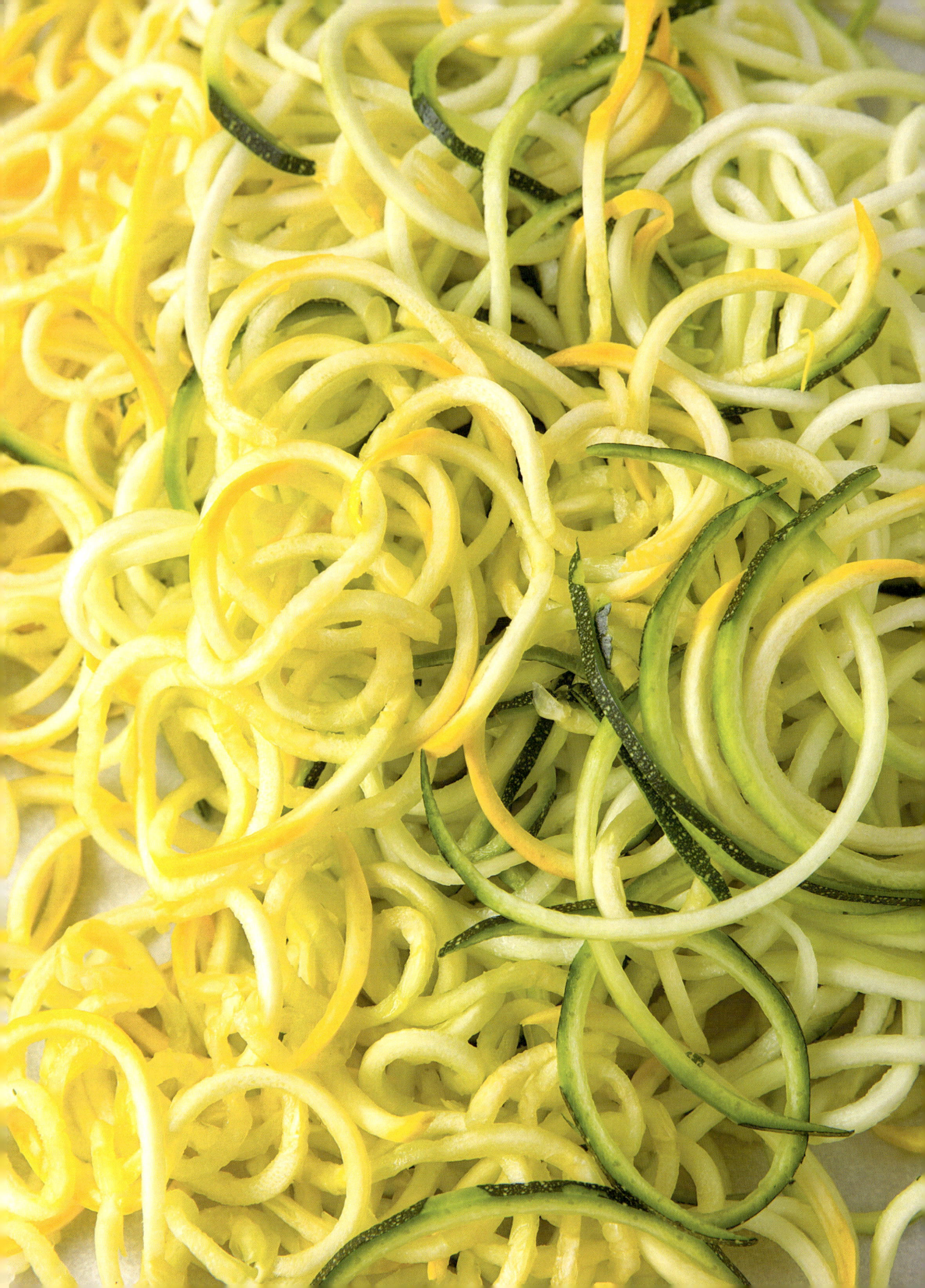

THE PERFECT ROASTED CHICKEN

Everyone should have this basic roasted chicken in their culinary repertoire.
Simple yet delicious, a roast chicken is beloved in so many cultures, and the distinctive smell
of a bird cooking in the oven just evokes a welcoming feeling of comfort and home. Once you have
mastered this basic technique, you can play around with flavors, rubs and butters and create a
different taste every time you cook it. It goes with ALL the other vegetables, grains and sauces
in this book and it's equally good served cold the next day! The Root Vegetable Medley will easily
make you a fan of these underground "gems." The Roast Vegetable Compote is one of my own
personal, time-honored dishes both for teaching cooking skills and making great flavors.

Make Hot and Fresh
Medley of Roasted Root Vegetables, Balsamic
Vinegar, Roast Vegetable Compote
Makes 4-6 Servings

Serve the Next Day Hot
Makes 1 Serving

The Perfect Roasted Chicken

1 each 4-4½ lbs chicken,
  giblets removed

Salt and pepper
Cooking twine
4 Tbsp olive oil

Preheat the oven to 375°F.

Rinse chicken thoroughly inside and out with cold running water. Dry thoroughly inside and out with paper toweling. Season the chicken inside and out with salt and pepper and rub the outside of the chicken with the oil. Truss the chicken, tying the legs together with kitchen string, and tuck the wing tips under the back.

Place the chicken, breast side down, on a V-shaped rack in a roasting pan. Roast for 20 minutes. Turn the chicken on its side and roast for 20 minutes longer. Turn the chicken on its other side and roast for another 20 minutes. Turn the chicken breast side up and roast until a digital-read thermometer inserted into the thickest part of a thigh registers 165-170°F, approximately 25-35 minutes longer, for a total roasting time of approximately 1½ hours.

Transfer the chicken to a warmed platter. Let rest for 5-10 minutes before carving.

With a boning knife, cut the two halves of the chicken away from the central carcass. Separate the breast from the thigh and leg and split the breast in half. Separate the thigh and leg.

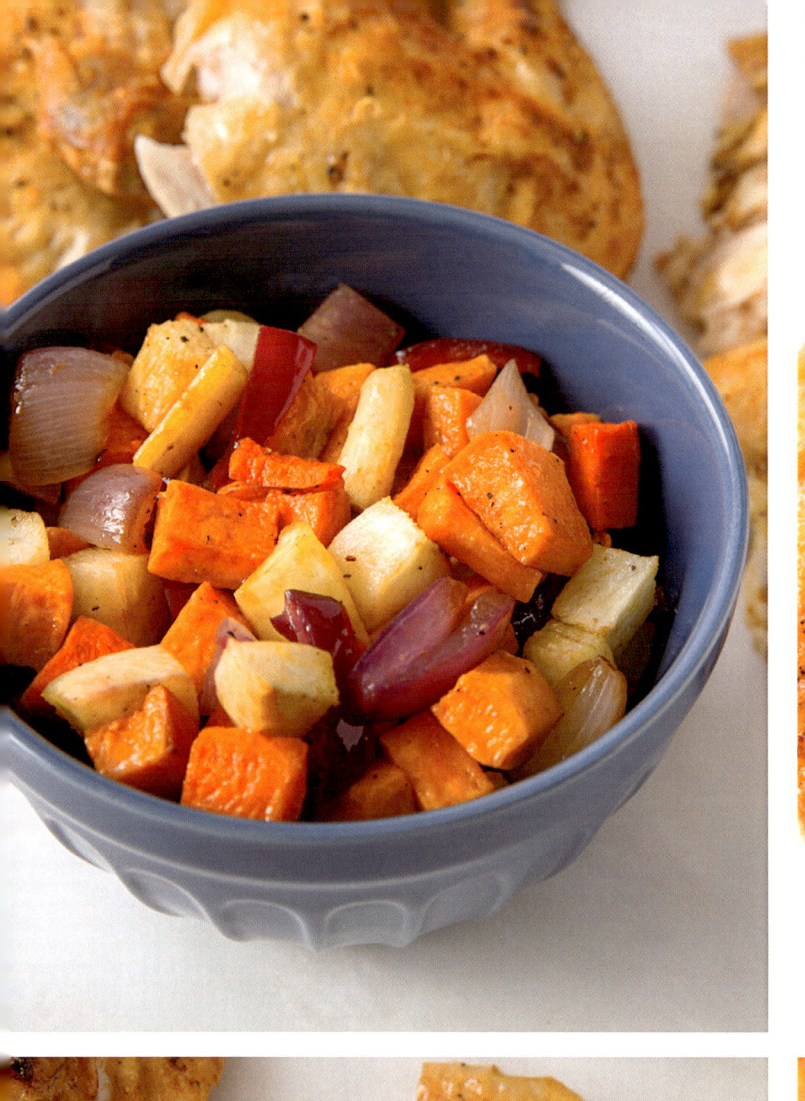
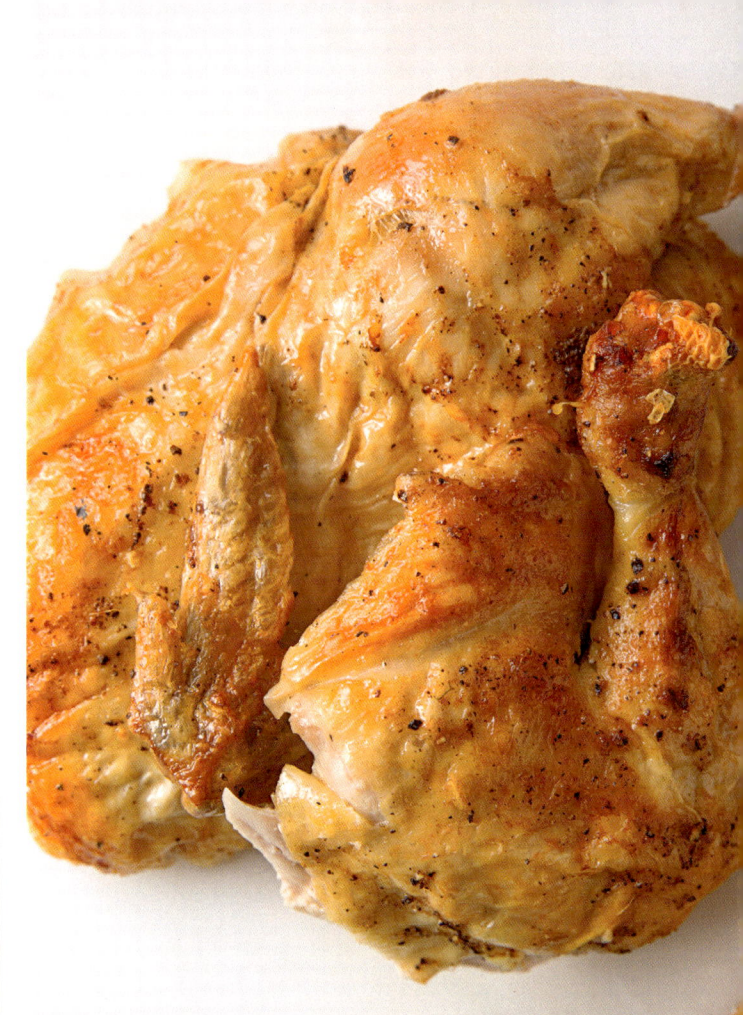
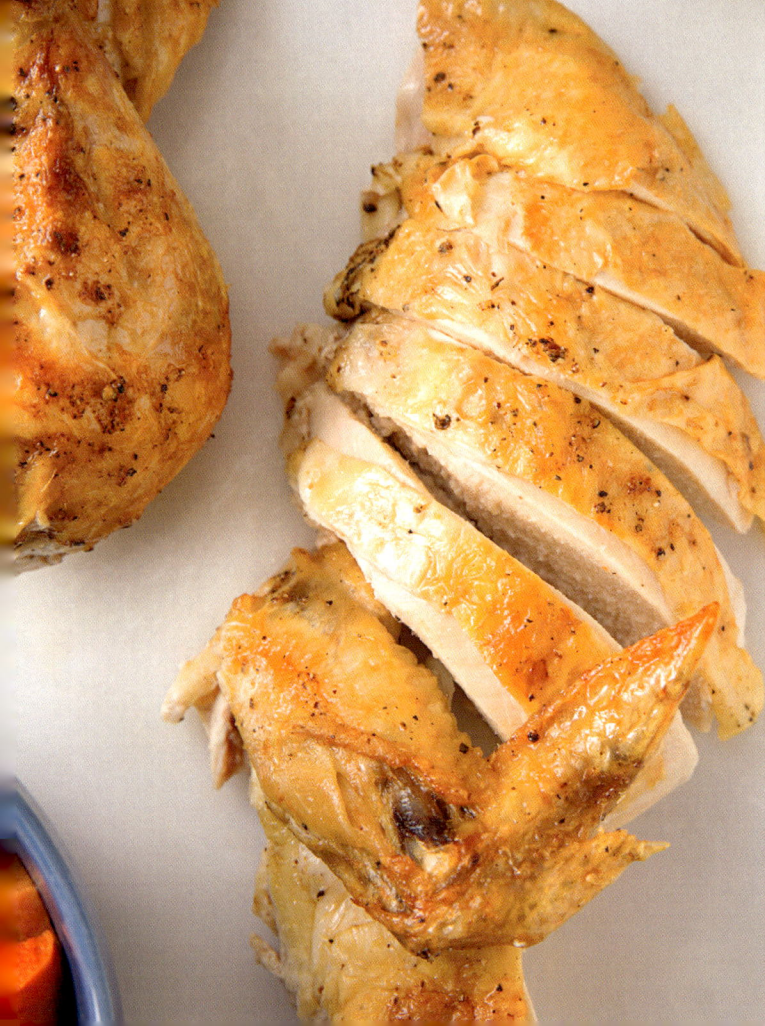
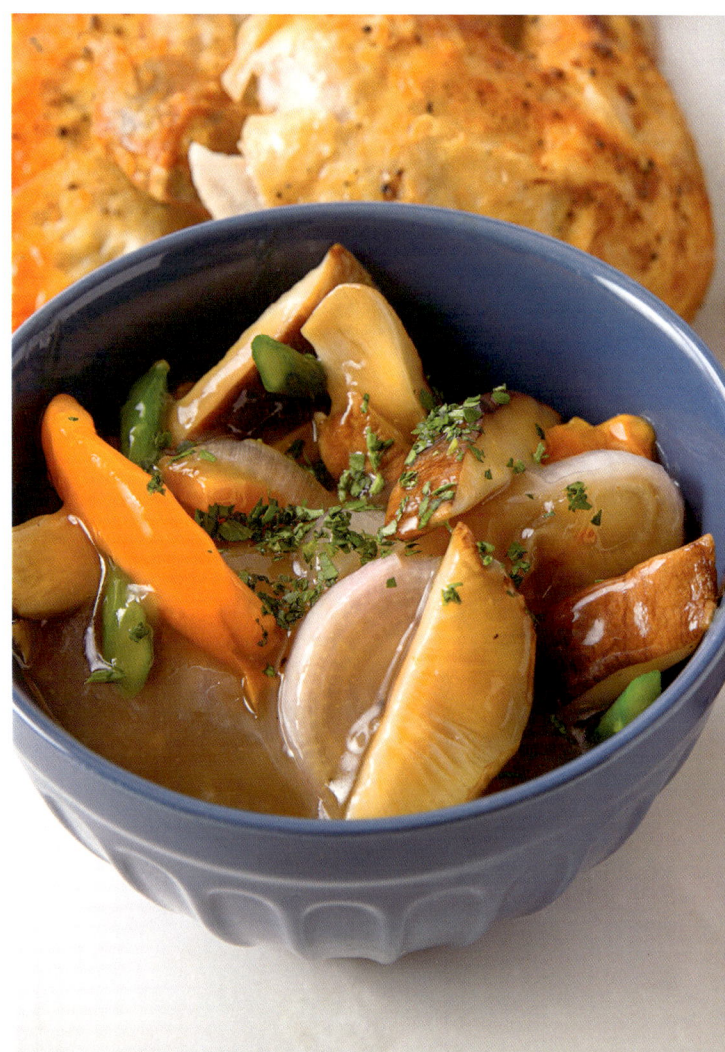

Medley of Roasted Root Vegetables

1 large red onion
¼ cup olive oil
Salt and pepper
2 lbs assorted root
   vegetables, such
    as carrots, turnips,
    parsnips or yams
2 Tbsp balsamic vinegar

Preheat oven to 375°F.

Split the onion in half, then brush the cut side with olive oil and season with salt and pepper. Place cut side down on a sheet pan and place in oven. Cook for 25-35 minutes until soft to the touch. Remove and let cool. Remove the outer layer of the onion and cut into large ½-inch dice.

Peel all root vegetables and cut into ½-inch cubes. Toss with just enough olive oil to coat, sprinkle with salt and pepper and lay out on sheet pan. **NOTE:** It is best to keep root vegetables separated and roast them individually. Roast 10-12 minutes until almost cooked through. Remove from the oven and immediately coat with balsamic vinegar. Set aside and let cool.

Just prior to serving, toss the root vegetables together with the red onion. Lay them out on a sheet pan and reheat in oven for 2-3 minutes. Remove and serve immediately.

Roast Vegetable Compote

¼ cup olive oil

1 large bunch asparagus, woody ends removed, cut in 6-inch lengths

2 large red bell peppers, stemmed and seeded

6 medium shallots, whole

6 oz Shiitake mushrooms, stemmed

1 cup beef stock

1 Tbsp arrowroot, diluted with water

2 Tbsp fresh tarragon, stemmed and chopped

Salt and pepper

Preheat oven to 375°F.

Cut, coat with olive oil, season and roast each vegetable according to the chart below.

Asparagus, medium 6-inch lengths	8-10 minutes
Red Bell Pepper laid flat	8-12 minutes
Shallots whole, unpeeled, covered	15-20 minutes
Shiitake Mushrooms whole, stemmed	7-10 minutes

When cooled, cut the asparagus and bell peppers into ½-inch lengths. Peel the shallot and thinly slice. Cut the Shiitakes into ½-inch dice. Set aside. In a medium saucepot, add the beef stock. Bring to a boil and thicken with the arrowroot. Add the asparagus, bell pepper, Shiitake mushrooms, shallot and tarragon and bring to a simmer. Remove from heat and add seasonings. Serve immediately. Makes about 3 cups

To Assemble

Serve the root vegetable medley, and top with 1 piece of chicken breast, and either a leg or a thigh. Equally portion the vegetable compote on top of the chicken. Serve immediately.

SERVE THE NEXT DAY HOT

½ cup Roasted Root Vegetables

4-5 oz Perfect Roasted Chicken

½ cup Roasted Vegetable Compote

Place vegetables in a microwave-proof plastic container, add chicken and cover with compote. When ready to eat, sprinkle with 1 Tbsp water, loosely place the lid on and reheat for 3-4 minutes or until hot all the way through.

CRISPY SKIN CHICKEN

Leave the skin on the chicken! You get far more flavor and nutrition with the skin on. It's hard to find boneless, skin on chicken breast. You can debone them yourself or cook them bone in which will add a few more minutes of cooking time. Tomatillo salsas are my favorite. I like the more peeled, acidic flavor profile they offer and are better cooked as in the salsa here. Supermarkets now offer peeled, seeded and cubed butternut squash to speed up your prep time but if your knife skills are still in need of improvement I encourage you to buy the squash whole and practice, practice, practice. If you don't like the taste of cilantro, simply leave it out.

Make Hot and Fresh	**Serve The Next Day Cold**
Tomatillo Salsa, Brown Rice with Garlic and Pine Nuts, Roasted Butternut Squash	Bed of Mixed Greens
Makes 4 Servings	*Makes 1 Serving*

Tomatillo Salsa

2 dried Guajillo chilies, stemmed and seeded

8 oz tomatillos

1 small onion, sliced about ⅛-inch

2 cloves garlic, unpeeled

1-2 Tbsp olive oil

Salt and pepper

1-2 limes

2 Tbsp cilantro, stemmed and chopped

Preheat oven to 350°F.

Place the chilies on a sheet pan and toast them in the oven for about 2-3 minutes. Do not leave them in too long or this will create acrid smoke in the room. Rehydrate them in 1 pint of very hot water for about 20 minutes, or until soft. Drain the chilies.

Remove the outer leaves from the tomatillos, rinse under warm water to remove the sticky film, dry with paper towels and cut in half. Place the sliced onion, tomatillos, and garlic on a small sheet pan. Lightly coat with olive oil and sprinkle with salt and pepper. Place in the oven and roast for 10-15 minutes until the onions and garlic are soft to the touch. Remove and let cool.

Peel the garlic. Add the chilies, onion, tomatillos and garlic to the blender or food processor and blend well. Juice the limes into the sauce, half a lime at a time, mixing after each addition to taste. Mix in the cilantro. Taste and adjust the seasonings, adding salt, if needed. Makes about 2 cups

Brown Rice with Garlic and Pine Nuts

1 Tbsp olive oil
1 shallot, minced
1 clove garlic, minced
1 cup brown rice
3 cups chicken stock
Salt and pepper, to taste
2 Tbsp toasted pine nuts
2 Tbsp minced Italian
   parsley

Heat a medium saucepot on medium heat. When hot, add the olive oil, shallot and garlic. Cook until soft, about 1 minute. Add the rice and stir to blend. Add the chicken stock, salt and pepper and stir just enough to loosen the rice. Bring to a boil, reduce to a simmer and cover. Cook approximately 40-45 minutes or until all liquid is absorbed. Remove from the heat and stir in the pine nuts and Italian parsley. Leave covered until ready to serve. Makes about 3 cups

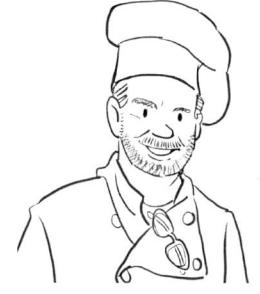

Don't give up on whole grains. Any whole grain that takes more than thirty minutes to cook may need adjusting on time and liquid from the packager's specifications.

Roasted Butternut Squash

½ butternut squash, peeled, seeded and cut into ½-inch cubes

1 Tbsp olive oil or to coat
Salt and pepper

Preheat oven to 350°F.

Place all the ingredients in a mixing bowl and toss to coat. Lay out the squash on a sheet pan without stacking and place in the oven. Cook for about 15 minutes, or until tender to the bite. Remove and let cool.

Crispy Skin Chicken

4 each 5-7 oz chicken breasts, skin on, deboned

Salt and pepper
1 Tbsp olive oil

Preheat the oven to 350°F.

Rinse and dry the chicken, then season with salt and pepper. Heat a large skillet on high heat. When very hot, add the oil, then the chicken. Cook until the skin is well-browned, about 4-5 minutes. Turn the chicken over and place in the oven for about 18-22 minutes, or until very firm to the touch. The internal temperature should be about 160°F. Remove and serve.

SERVE THE NEXT DAY COLD
Bed of Mixed Greens

To Assemble

Large handful mixed greens

¼ cup any roasted and salted nuts or seeds

4-6 oz Crispy Skin Chicken, sliced thin

½ cup Brown Rice with Garlic and Pine Nuts

¾ cup Roasted Butternut Squash

¼ cup Tomatillo Salsa

In separate travel containers, pack the greens; the nuts; the chicken, rice and squash; and lastly, the salsa. When ready to serve, place all ingredients in a serving bowl and toss together.

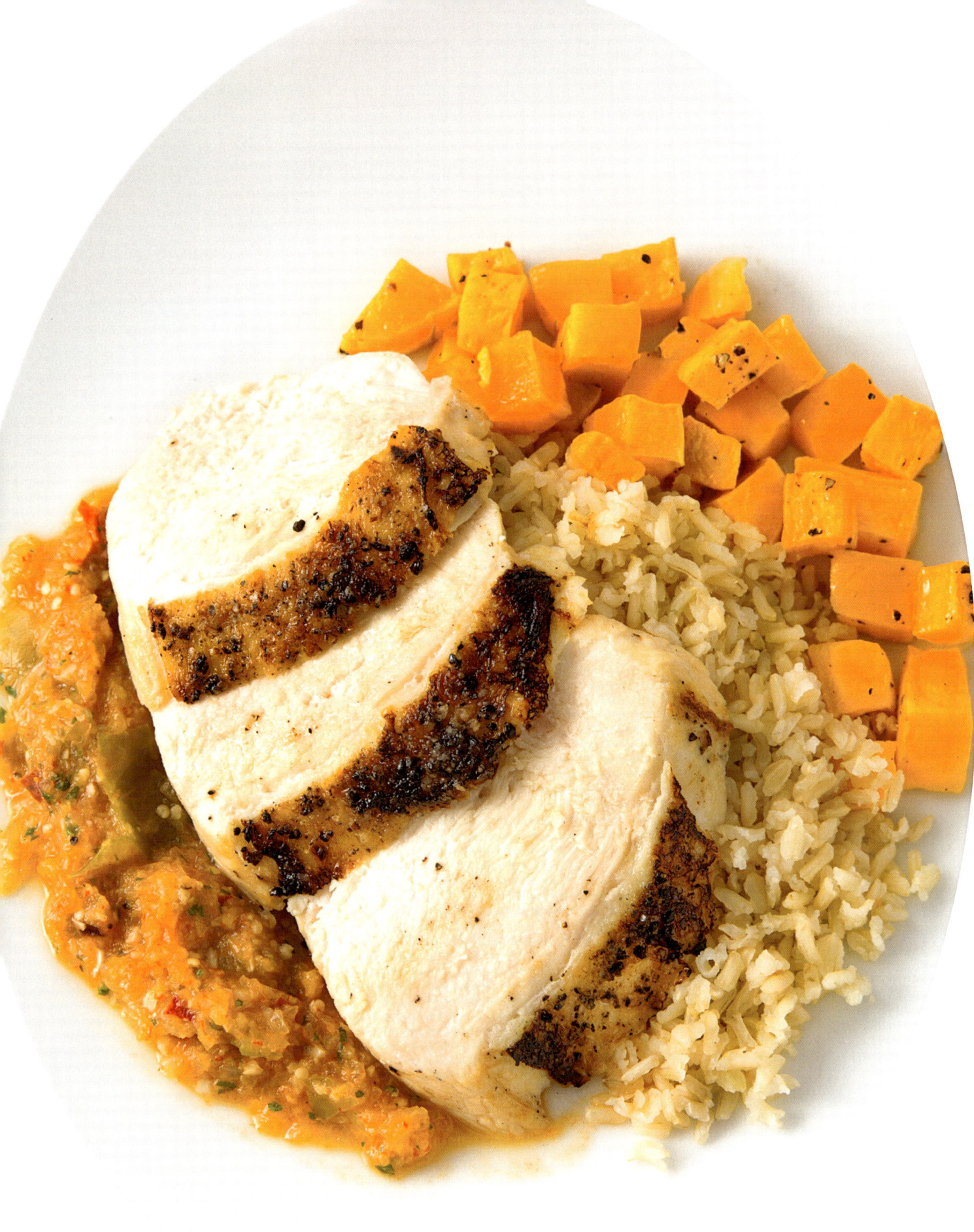

CHILI RUBBED BREAST OF CHICKEN

Chicken breasts come in varying sizes, so one of the techniques I frequently use is to flatten them, which results in a very quick and even cooking time on the stove. If you don't own a meat tenderizer, just place the breasts between two sheets of plastic wrap and use a sturdy skillet to flatten them. This Black Bean Relish has been one of my go to recipes for the past 25 years, served both hot and cold so don't be afraid to make extra and use often with other dishes. Make certain to use organic polenta.

Make Hot and Fresh
Black Bean Relish, Creamy Polenta
Makes 4 Servings

Serve The Next Day Hot
Makes 1 Serving

Black Bean Relish

⅓ cup olive oil
1½ cups assorted colored bell peppers, diced
1 Anaheim pepper, seeded and diced
1 cup diced yellow onions
2 cloves garlic, minced
2 cups canned black beans, drained and rinsed
1 cup corn kernels
1-2 Tbsp chili powder
3-4 Tbsp lime juice
Salt and pepper

In a large sauté pan, add 1 Tbsp olive oil and bring to high heat. Add the peppers, onions and garlic and sauté for approximately 2 minutes, or until softened. Transfer to a large mixing bowl. Add the black beans and corn and mix thoroughly. Add the chili powder, lime juice, salt and pepper and mix. Add the remaining olive oil and toss well. Taste and adjust seasonings.

When ready to serve, place all ingredients back in the sauté pan and heat the relish over medium heat until warmed through. Makes about 4 cups

Creamy Polenta

4 cups water
Large pinch salt
1 cup organic Italian-style polenta
⅓ cup grated Asiago cheese
2 Tbsp unsalted butter

In a large saucepot, bring the water and salt to a full boil. Add the polenta to the water in a thin steady stream, while stirring continuously with a high temperature rubber spatula or wooden spoon. When all the polenta has been added, reduce the heat to a simmer.

Continue cooking for approximately 10-12 minutes, stirring often, until the polenta is cooked and soft and creamy to the bite. Remove the pot from the heat and add the Asiago cheese and butter. This is the basic technique for cooking all polenta. Keep covered and warm until ready to serve.

NOTE: Extra polenta can be spread on a sheet pan, covered and chilled. To serve the next day, cut in any shape you desire and reheat. These are Polenta Cakes.

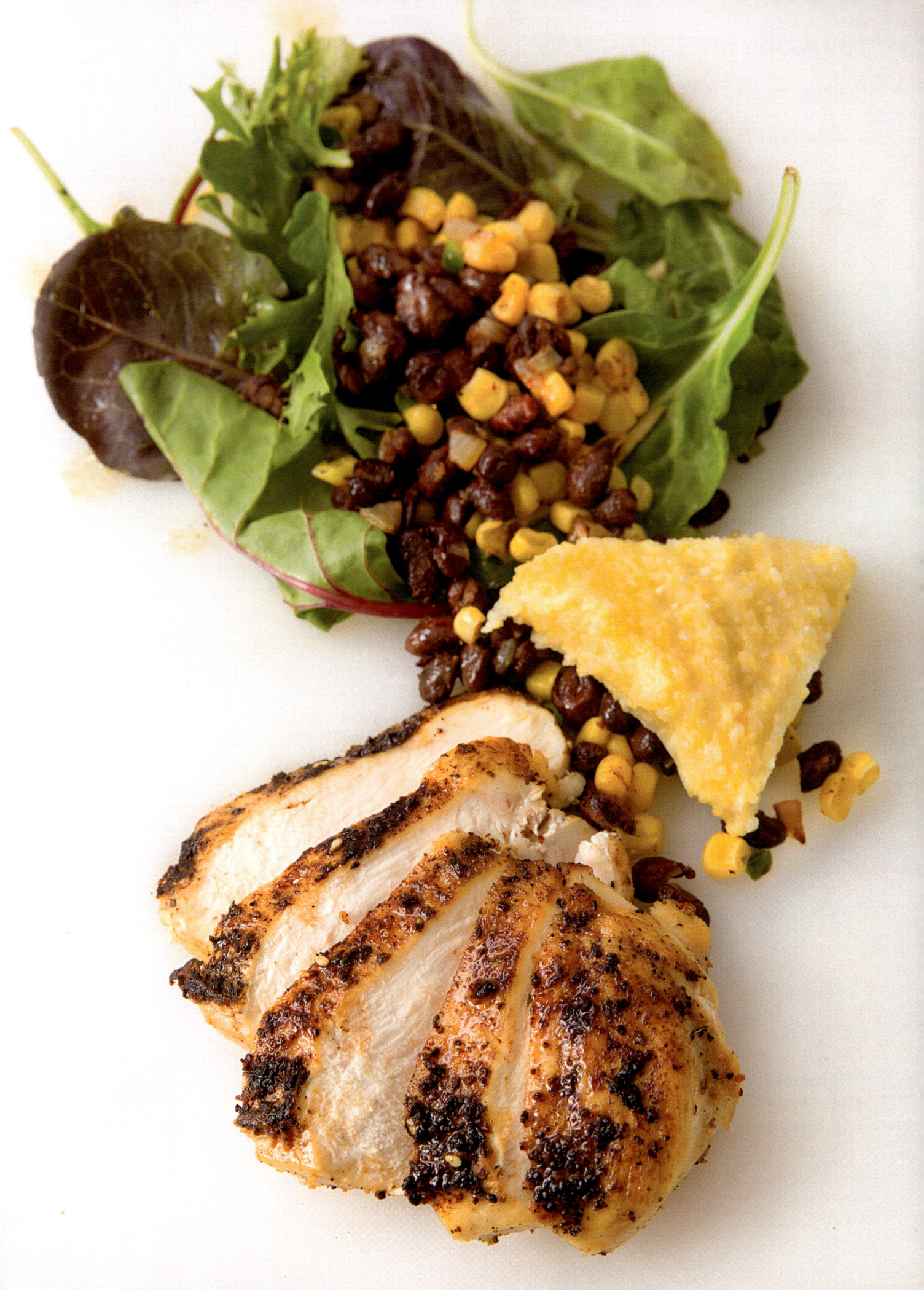

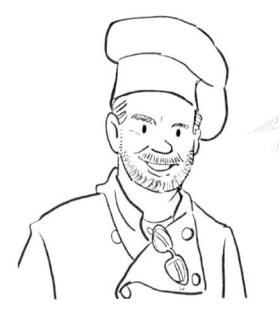

This chicken dish calls for Mexican oregano, which is different from Greek oregano. Both offer very different flavors and don't always interchange, so I recommend that you have both on hand in your spice drawer.

Chili Rubbed Breast of Chicken

4 each 5-7 oz chicken breasts, skin on and deboned

2 Tbsp chili powder

2 tsp dried whole Mexican oregano

½ tsp salt
½ tsp garlic powder
½ tsp onion powder
2 Tbsp olive oil

Lay the chicken breasts on a clean work surface, cover with plastic wrap and using the flat side of a meat tenderizer, flatten chicken to about ¾-inch thick. On a large plate or sheet pan, lay out the chicken breasts. In a small bowl, combine all the dried seasonings together. Sprinkle the spice mixture over both sides of the breasts. Lightly coat with some of the olive oil. Cover and refrigerate for 30 minutes or up to 3 hours.

Heat a large skillet and add the remaining olive oil. Add the chicken breasts to the skillet without crowding or stacking. Reduce heat to medium and cook approximately 6-8 minutes until golden brown. Turn the chicken over and continue to cook until very firm and springy to the touch, another 6-8 minutes. The internal temperature should be about 160°F. Set aside and keep warm.

To Assemble

Serve the chicken topped with the Black Bean Relish, and with Creamy Polenta.

SERVE THE NEXT DAY HOT

To Assemble

3 oz cold Polenta Cake
5 oz chili Rubbed Breast of Chicken, sliced thin

½ cup Black Bean Relish

Place the polenta in a microwave-proof plastic container, top with chicken and cover with relish. Just prior to serving, sprinkle with 1 Tbsp water, loosely place the lid on and reheat for 3-4 minutes or until hot all the way through.

ASIAN CHICKEN SKEWERS

Visiting your local Asian store can be an exciting shopping experience and I highly recommend it! The Tandoori Paste and Chinese Chili Paste used here can be found at most Asian markets. Both of these concentrated pastes contribute big bold flavor to these chicken skewers, which are happy to sit marinating in the fridge for a day, and a great choice for a dish that can be made well in advance.

Make Hot and Fresh
Tandoori Noodles
Makes 4 Servings

Serve The Next Day Cold
Makes 1 Serving

Tandoori Noodles

2 Tbsp soy sauce

2 Tbsp raw honey

1 Tbsp minced fresh
  ginger

1-2 garlic cloves, minced

3 Tbsp Tandoori paste

2 Tbsp minced cilantro

1 Tbsp sesame oil

2 Tbsp fresh lemon juice

Salt

6 oz any Asian style
  noodle, preferably rice
  noodles

¼ cup pistachios, roughly
  chopped

In a large mixing bowl, combine well the first 8 ingredients. Set aside or cover and refrigerate. The sauce will keep for 3-4 days.

When ready to serve, bring a large pot of water to boil and add salt. Add the noodles and cook according to the package directions. When done, drain well and add to the sauce. Just prior to serving, top with the chopped pistachios.

When making any kind of skewers or kebobs, don't miss the essential step of pre-soaking the thin wooden bamboo skewers in cold water for a few minutes – this stops them from burning when the skewers are cooking on the grill.

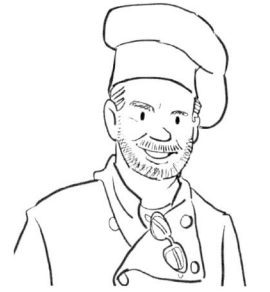

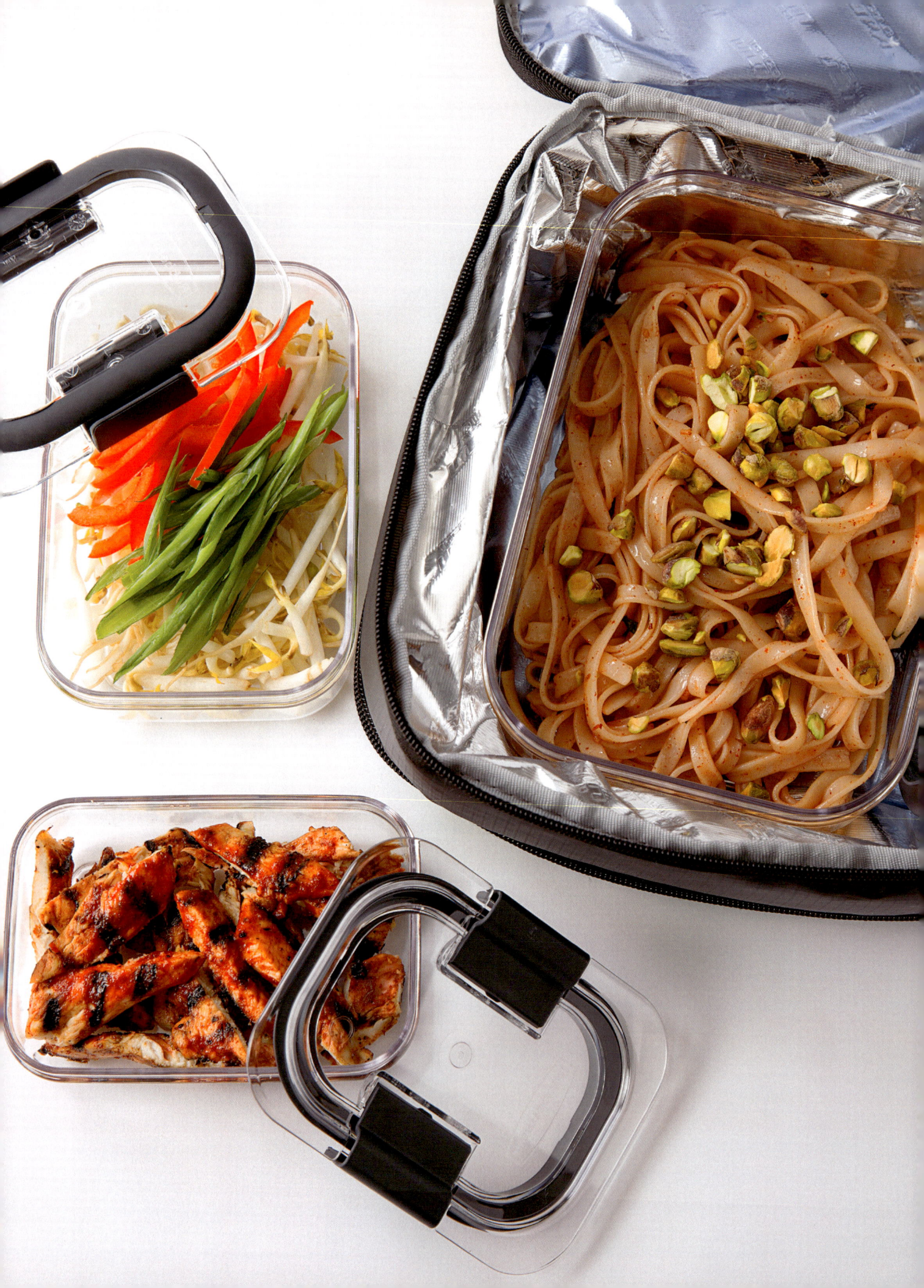

Asian Chicken Skewers

Bamboo skewers
1¼ lbs chicken breast,
  boneless and skinless

3 Tbsp Tandoori paste
3 Tbsp lime juice
2 Tbsp raw honey
2 Tbsp fish sauce
1 Tbsp Chinese chili
  paste

1-2 Tbsp olive oil

Soak 20 bamboo skewers in cold water for about 15 minutes. Slice the chicken into long, thin pieces about ¼-inch thick. Thread the chicken onto the bamboo skewers.

In a small mixing bowl, combine the remaining ingredients, except the olive oil, and blend very well. Thoroughly coat the skewers with the marinade. Set aside or cover and refrigerate until ready to cook, from 30 minutes to overnight.

Heat a grill on medium heat.

Remove any excess marinade from the skewers. Brush the olive oil onto the skewers. Place the skewers on the grill and cook for about 2-3 minutes on each side, or until very firm and springy to the touch.

Serve the noodles topped with the skewers. Serve immediately.

SERVE THE NEXT DAY COLD

To Assemble

1 cup Tandoori Noodles
4-5 oz Asian Chicken
  Skewers, bamboo
  skewers removed

¼ cup bean sprouts
2 green onions, julienned
¼ cup julienned red bell
  pepper

Assemble the noodles and chicken skewers in a travel container, placing the three raw vegetables in a separate container. When ready to serve, toss with the raw vegetables.

MOLE-RUBBED CHICKEN

A classic Mole is a traditional Mexican sauce, but here we are using its flavors to create a dry rub seasoning. For convenience, you can also find pre-made Mole spice rubs for sale at specialty food stores. Turbinado sugar is pure cane sugar extract, with a light brown color and a slightly more subtle flavor than regular brown sugar. Cumin Lime Rice is a favorite in our house and it complements any Mexican or Southwestern entrée. Grilling the fruit for the Mojo caramelizes the fruit and elevates the flavor profile.

Make Hot and Fresh
Grilled Fruit Mojo, Cumin Lime Rice,
Grilled Summer Squash
Makes 4 Servings

Serve The Next Day Cold
Lettuce Wraps
Makes 1 Serving

Mole Rub

2 Tbsp cocoa powder
2 Tbsp turbinado sugar
2 Tbsp salt
1 Tbsp pumpkin seeds, toasted

2 Tbsp roasted peanuts
1 Tbsp mild chili powder
1 Tbsp ancho chili powder

½ tsp ground ginger
½ tsp ground anise
½ tsp ground cinnamon
2 whole cloves
1 tsp ground coriander
½ tsp ground dry oregano

½ tsp ground dry marjoram

Pinch ground allspice

Combine all ingredients in a food processor and process to a powder. Set aside. Makes about ¾ cup

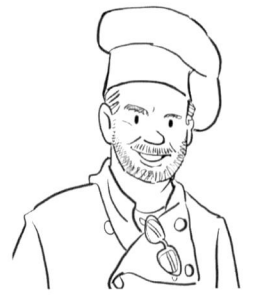

All chile powders are not created equal! Always taste a little bit to see how hot your particular jar of spice is — that way you can adjust the amounts you add accordingly.

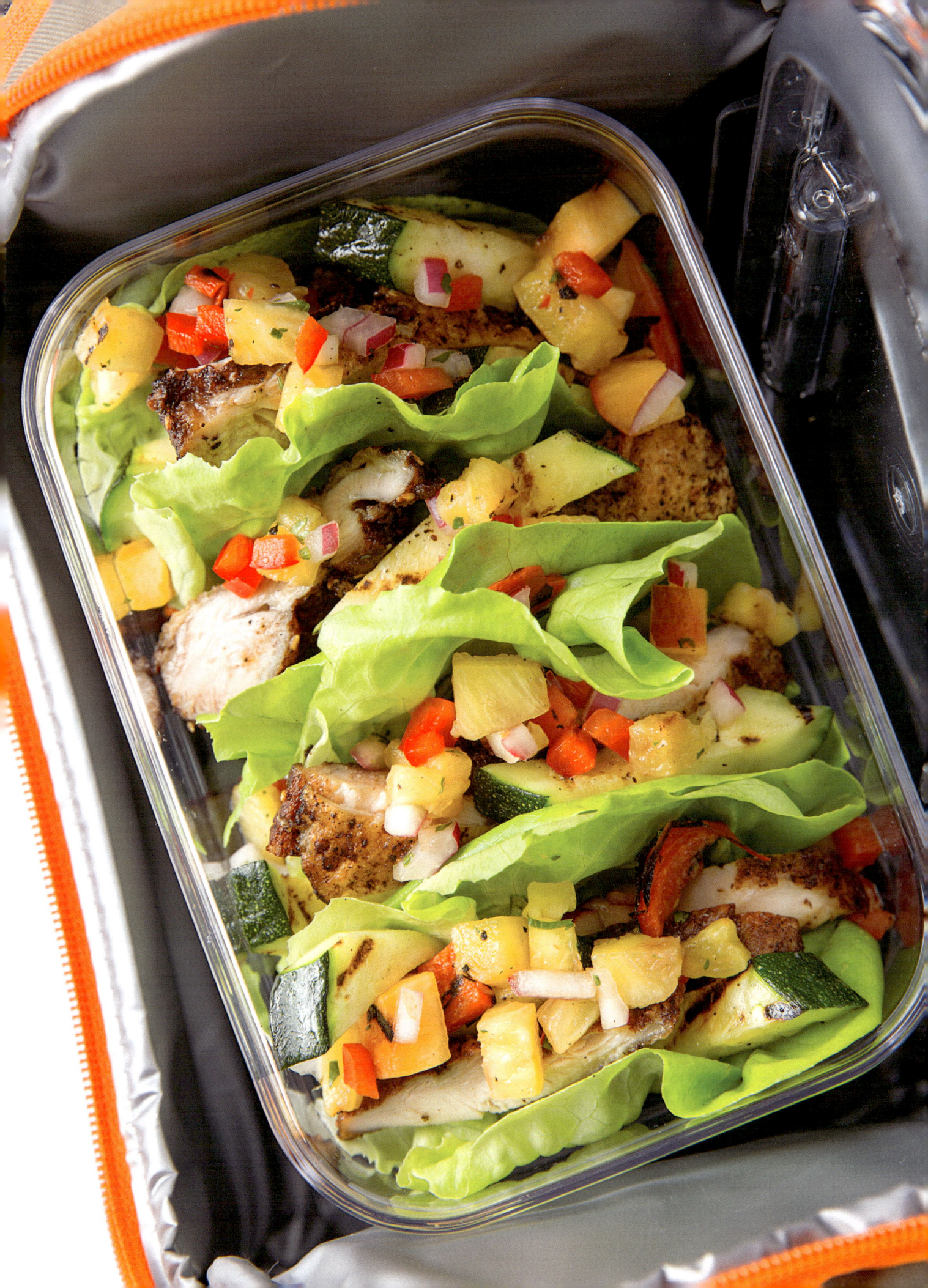

Cumin Lime Rice

1 Tbsp olive oil
½ small yellow onion, minced
1 stalk celery, washed and minced
1 small carrot, minced
1 clove garlic, minced
1 tsp ground cumin
1 bay leaf
¾ cup long grain brown rice
2¼ cups chicken broth
Zest and juice of 1 lime
Salt and pepper

Heat a medium saucepot. When hot, add the olive oil. Place the onion, celery and carrot in the pot, reduce the heat to medium and sauté for about 1½ - 2 minutes, or until soft. Add the garlic, cumin, bay leaf and the rice and stir to blend completely.

Add the chicken broth, lime zest, juice and seasonings and stir once or twice, just enough to loosen the rice. Bring to a boil, cover with a tight-fitting lid and reduce the heat to a simmer. Cook for approximately 40-45 minutes or until all the liquid is absorbed. Remove from the heat and leave covered for at least 5-10 minutes before serving. Makes about 2 cups

Grilled Fruit Mojo

2-3 Tbsp melted coconut oil
3 each ½-inch thick slices peeled pineapple
Optional, 3 apricots, split and seeded
½ red bell pepper, stemmed, split and seeded
1 small red onion, cut in ½-inch thick slices
½ tsp chili powder
2 Tbsp minced cilantro
1-2 Tbsp lime juice, to taste
3-4 Tbsp orange juice
Salt

Heat a grill or indoor grill plate on high heat.

Using the coconut oil, brush all sides of the fruits and vegetables. Cook the pineapple for about 90 seconds on each side, then remove and let cool. Cook the apricots, if using, for about 2 minutes, on the cut side only. Remove and let cool. Cook the bell pepper and onion for about 3-4 minutes on each side or until soft. Remove and let cool.

When cooled, cut all the fruits and vegetables into ¼-inch dice.

Place fruit and vegetables in a mixing bowl; add the chili powder, cilantro and mix in the fruit juices. Add salt and taste and adjust seasonings, adding more juices if needed. Serve immediately or place in the refrigerator up to 4 hours. Makes about 2 cups

Grilled Summer Squash

1 medium zucchini
1 medium yellow squash
1 tsp olive oil
Salt and pepper

Heat a grill or indoor grill plate on high heat.

Trim and cut the squashes on the bias about a ¼-inch thick. Lay the slices on a sheet pan, brush both sides with oil and season with salt and pepper. Place the squash on the grill, cook for 3-4 minutes per side, or until bendable to the touch. Remove and serve, or let cool.

Mole Rubbed Chicken Thighs

8 each 6 to 8 oz boneless
   chicken thighs
3-4 Tbsp vegetable oil
¼ cup mole rub

Rinse the chicken and pat dry with paper towel. Brush the vegetable oil onto the chicken and rub the Mole Rub evenly over it, patting in on all sides. Cover and refrigerate for at least 30 minutes or up to 1 day.

When ready to cook, heat a grill or indoor grill plate on high heat.

When hot, place the thighs on the grill and reduce the heat to medium-low and close the lid of the grill , or cover with a domed lid. Cook, turning as necessary, for approximately 12-15 minutes, or until the thighs are springy to the touch. Remove and transfer to a cutting board and slice on a 45˚ bias in approximately ¼-inch slices.

SERVE THE NEXT DAY COLD
Lettuce Wraps

To Assemble

4 oz Mole Rubbed
   Chicken, chopped

½ cup Cumin Lime Rice

⅓ cup Grilled Summer
   Squash, julienned

⅓ cup Grilled Fruit Mojo

4 large Bibb lettuce
   leaves, washed and
   dried

Green onions to garnish

Pack each item separately in its own travel container. When ready to eat, place small portions of each item onto the lettuce leaves, wrap and serve.

> When working with citrus juice, as in the fruit mojo, consider it a seasoning that can be tasted and adjusted accordingly, just like salt and pepper.

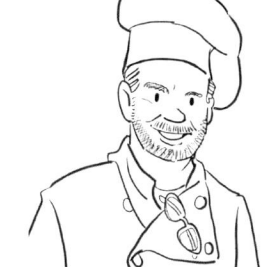

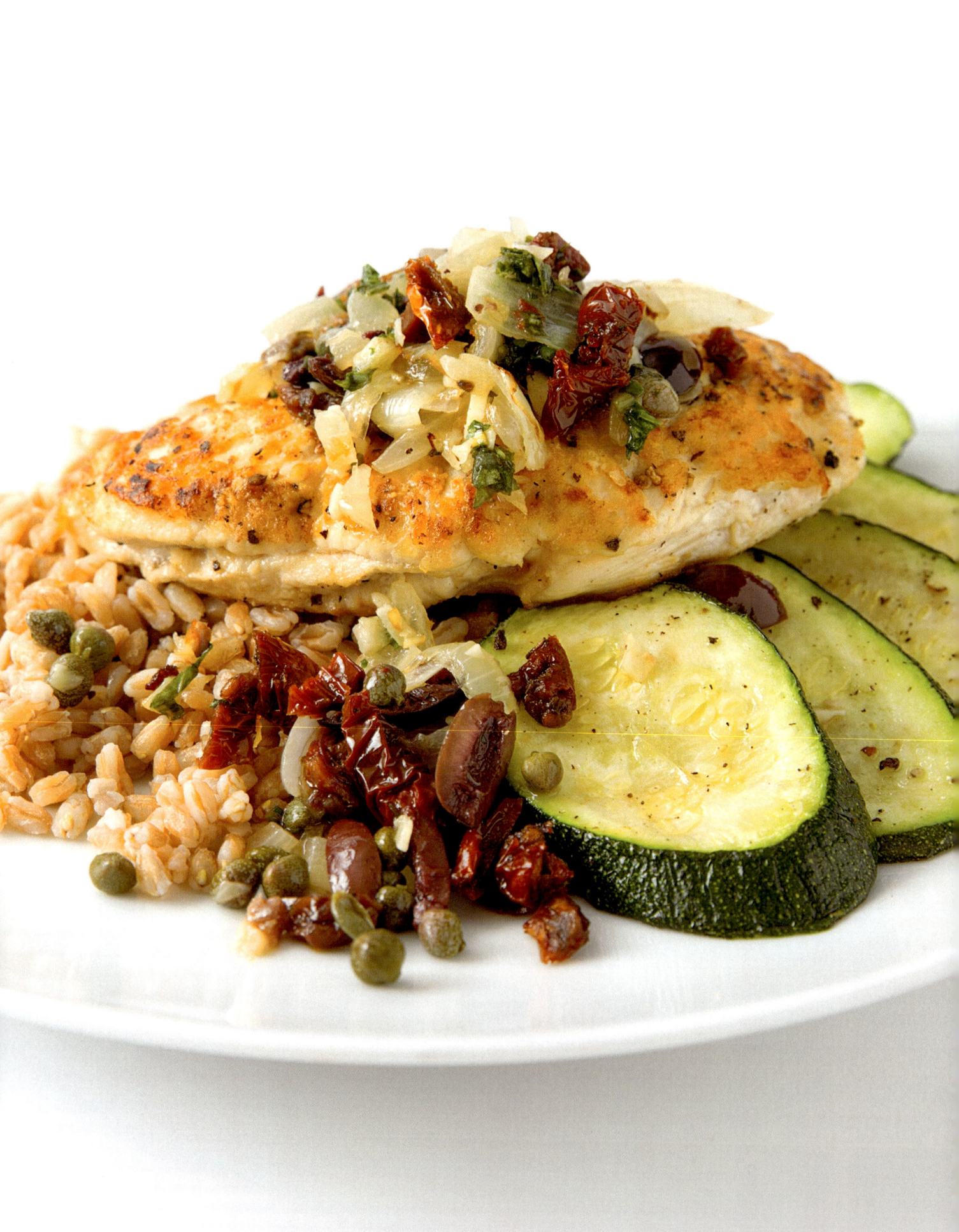

CHICKEN PUTTANESCA

Traditional Mediterranean flavors are bold, sunny and bright! Plus, the benefits of an authentic Mediterranean diet have been well-documented, being rich in cured, pickled and fresh vegetables, whole grains and plenty of olive oil. This is a truly iconic Italian recipe, and a great choice for a quick and delicious meal. It boasts a wonderful "umami" or earthy flavor profile, thanks to its abundance of tomatoes, olives, anchovies, garlic and capers. To save even more time, I have substituted the traditional canned tomatoes for oil-packed sun-dried tomatoes, which do not even need to be cooked, just warmed through. Farro is a classic Italian whole grain, readily available in natural food stores.

Make Hot and Fresh
Farro, Spaghetti Squash
Makes 4 Servings

Serve The Next Day Hot
Makes 1 Serving

Farro

3 cups water
Pinch salt
¾ cup farro

Bring the water and salt to a boil. Add the farro and stir once. Reduce to a simmer and cover. Cook for 15-30 minutes, checking for doneness every few minutes. Farro should be tender but chewy to the bite. Drain excess water and keep covered and warm until ready to serve. Makes about 1½ cups

Puttanesca Sauce

¼ cup olive oil
1 small onion, diced
3 cloves minced garlic
¼ cup oil-packed
   sun-dried tomatoes,
   julienned

½ cup pitted Kalamata
   olives, cut in half

2 Tbsp tomato paste
2 Tbsp drained capers
2 Tbsp minced anchovy
   fillets
2 Tbsp stemmed and
   sliced basil
Pinch red pepper flakes
Salt

Heat a medium skillet on medium high heat. When hot, add the olive oil, then add the onion and sauté for about 5-6 minutes, or until soft and lightly caramelized. Add the garlic and cook for an additional 20 seconds. Add the remaining ingredients and bring to heat. Remove, taste and adjust the seasonings. This type of Puttanesca is best served at room temperature. Makes about 2 cups

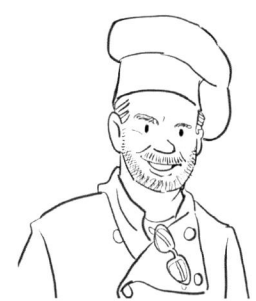

This Puttanesca Sauce is a very convenient weeknight supper dish, as it makes use of many Mediterranean pantry staples that you may always have on hand.

Sautéed Chicken Breasts

4 each 6 oz boneless
  skinless chicken breasts
Salt and pepper
1-2 Tbsp olive oil

Place a sheet of plastic wrap on a cutting board or worktable. Lay the chicken breasts on the plastic wrap about 2 inches apart. Lay another sheet of plastic wrap over the chicken breasts. With a meat cleaver or tenderizing hammer, gently flatten the chicken breasts to a thickness of about ½-inch. Unwrap and season the chicken breasts with the salt and pepper.

Heat a large skillet with 1 Tbsp of the olive oil. When very hot, add the chicken breasts. Reduce the heat to medium and cook on each side for 4-6 minutes, until the chicken is brown on each side and springs back to the touch. Remove the chicken to a warm platter.

Spaghetti Squash

1 spaghetti squash
Salt and pepper
Olive oil

Preheat oven to 350°F.

Cut squash in half, season with salt, pepper and olive oil, and place cut side up on a baking sheet. Roast for 40-45 minutes or until soft enough to push in the skin with your finger. Remove and let cool enough to handle.

Holding the squash half with a towel, use a fork or kitchen spoon to pull the cooked squash from the skin, so it resembles noodles, and season again to taste with salt and pepper. Cover and keep warm until ready to use.

SERVE THE NEXT DAY HOT

½ cup Farro
1 Sautéed Chicken
  Breast, sliced
¾ cup Spaghetti Squash
¼ cup Puttanesca Sauce

Place the Farro in a microwave-proof plastic container, top with Sautéed Chicken Breast, Spaghetti Squash, and Puttanesca Sauce. Sprinkle 1 Tbsp water on top, loosely place the lid on top then reheat for 3-4 minutes or until hot all the way through.

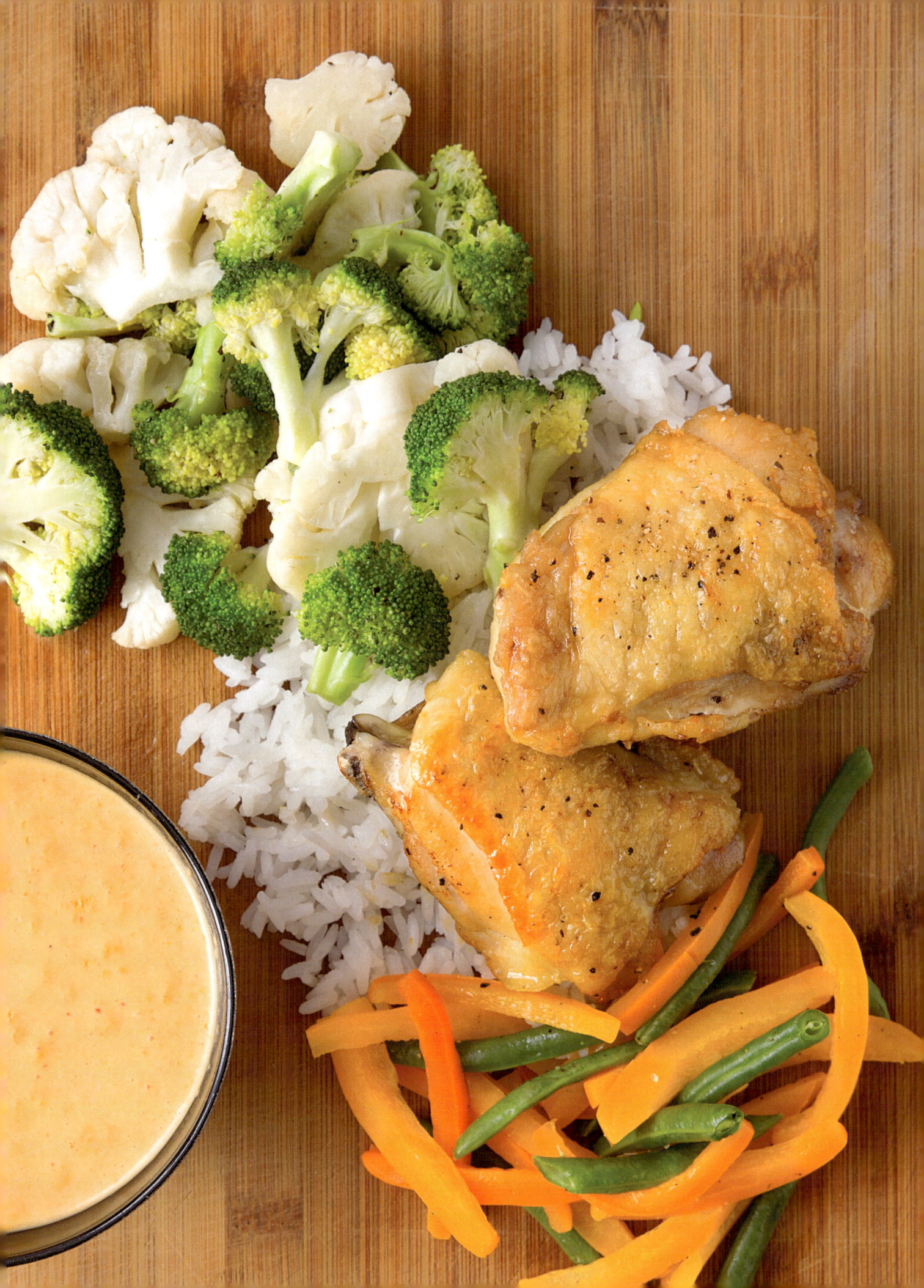

PAN ROASTED CHICKEN THIGHS

This curry coconut sauce is a wonderful base for any protein, and adds a distinct Asian flair to your meal, without adding refined sugar, which is all too often found in many traditional dishes from that part of the world. It only works hot so I've included a nice miso vinaigrette to serve the next day cold. I always prefer to use chicken thighs, as they are inexpensive, juicier and more flavorful than chicken breasts – plus they are also harder to overcook. The steamed vegetables will work beautifully with any dish, any time and can be made with a large variety of vegetables. Optional garnishes for the chicken include chopped fresh cilantro or Italian parsley, as well as chopped nuts or seeds, e.g., pecans, pumpkin seeds or cashews.

Make Hot and Fresh
Curry Coconut Sauce, Steamed Vegetable Medley, Jasmine Rice
Makes 4 Servings

Serve the Next Day Cold
Miso Vinaigrette and Mixed Greens
Makes 1 Serving

Curry Coconut Sauce

2 Tbsp olive oil

1 Tbsp peeled and chopped ginger

2 cloves garlic, chopped

1 small carrot, peeled and chopped

1 small onion, chopped

2 celery stalks, chopped

1-2 Tbsp red, yellow, or green curry paste

2 cups coconut milk

1-2 Tbsp fresh lime juice

Heat a medium-size saucepan on medium heat, and add the oil. Add the ginger, garlic, carrot, onion, and celery; cook until tender. Add the curry paste and cook for another minute. Watch carefully so it does not burn. Add the coconut milk, bring to a simmer and cook until the vegetables are tender. Transfer to a blender and purée.

Return the sauce to the saucepan and add the fresh lime juice. Keep warm until ready to serve. Makes about 3 cups

Pan Roasted Chicken Thighs

8 each 6 to 8 oz chicken thighs, bone in, skin on
Salt and pepper
1Tbsp olive oil

Preheat oven to 350°F.

Rinse the chicken and dry with paper towels. Season with salt and pepper. Heat a large skillet on high heat. When hot, add the olive oil, then the thighs, skin side down. Cook for 2-3 minutes or until the skin of the chicken is well-browned. Turn the thighs over, then place in the oven. Cook for about 20-25 minutes, until very firm to the touch and the internal temperature has reached 165°F. Remove and let cool. Remove the bone and cut chicken into thin ½-inch strips.

Jasmine Rice

1½ cups Jasmine rice, rinsed
2¼ cups cold water
Salt

Place all the ingredients in a medium saucepot and stir once to moisten rice. Do not stir again during the entire cooking process. Place on high heat and bring to a boil. Cover the saucepot with a tight-fitting lid and reduce the heat to a low simmer. Cook for approximately 25 minutes or until all the water is absorbed. Remove from heat and leave covered for at least 5-10 minutes before serving. Makes about 2½ cups

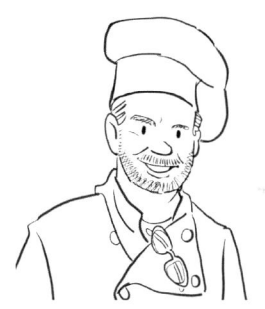

When making a classic vinaigrette, you can use any number of different vinegars, oils and emulsifiers. But whatever the flavor profile, there is one rule I always adhere to — when adding the oil, whip fast, and add slow!

Steamed Vegetable Medley

4 oz green beans, cut on
  a bias

1 red bell pepper,
  julienned

4 oz cauliflower, sliced
  very thin

4 oz broccoli, sliced very
  thin

Salt and pepper

Set up a steamer and bring to a boil. Place the vegetables in a steamer basket and sprinkle with salt and pepper. Cook for 3-4 minutes, or until all the vegetables are tender-crisp to the bite. Remove and serve immediately. If not serving immediately, place the vegetables in a bowl of ice water until cold, then drain and set aside.

NOTE: Optional garnishes for the chicken include ¼ cup chopped fresh cilantro or Italian parsley, as well as chopped nuts or seeds (e.g., pecans, pumpkin seeds or cashews).

SERVE THE NEXT DAY COLD
Miso Vinaigrette and Mixed Greens

Miso Vinaigrette

1 Serrano chili, stemmed,
  seeded and minced

1-2 Tbsp lime juice

2 Tbsp Miso paste, any
  color

2 Tbsp Tamari

2 Tbsp unseasoned rice
  vinegar

2 Tbsp toasted sesame
  oil

½ cup avocado, grape
  seed or olive oil

In a medium mixing bowl, combine all ingredients except the oils. Whisk together, and while continuing to whisk, slowly add the oil. Taste and adjust the seasonings. Keep covered and refrigerate until ready to serve. Makes about 1 cup

To Assemble

Large handful mixed
  greens

½ cup Jasmine Rice

5 oz Pan Roasted Chicken
  Thighs, sliced

½ cup Steamed Vegetable
  Medley

¼ cup Miso Vinaigrette
Optional garnishes

Place the greens and any optional garnishes in one travel container; the rice, chicken and vegetables in a second container; and the vinaigrette in a third. When ready to eat, place all the ingredients in a bowl, toss to coat and serve immediately.

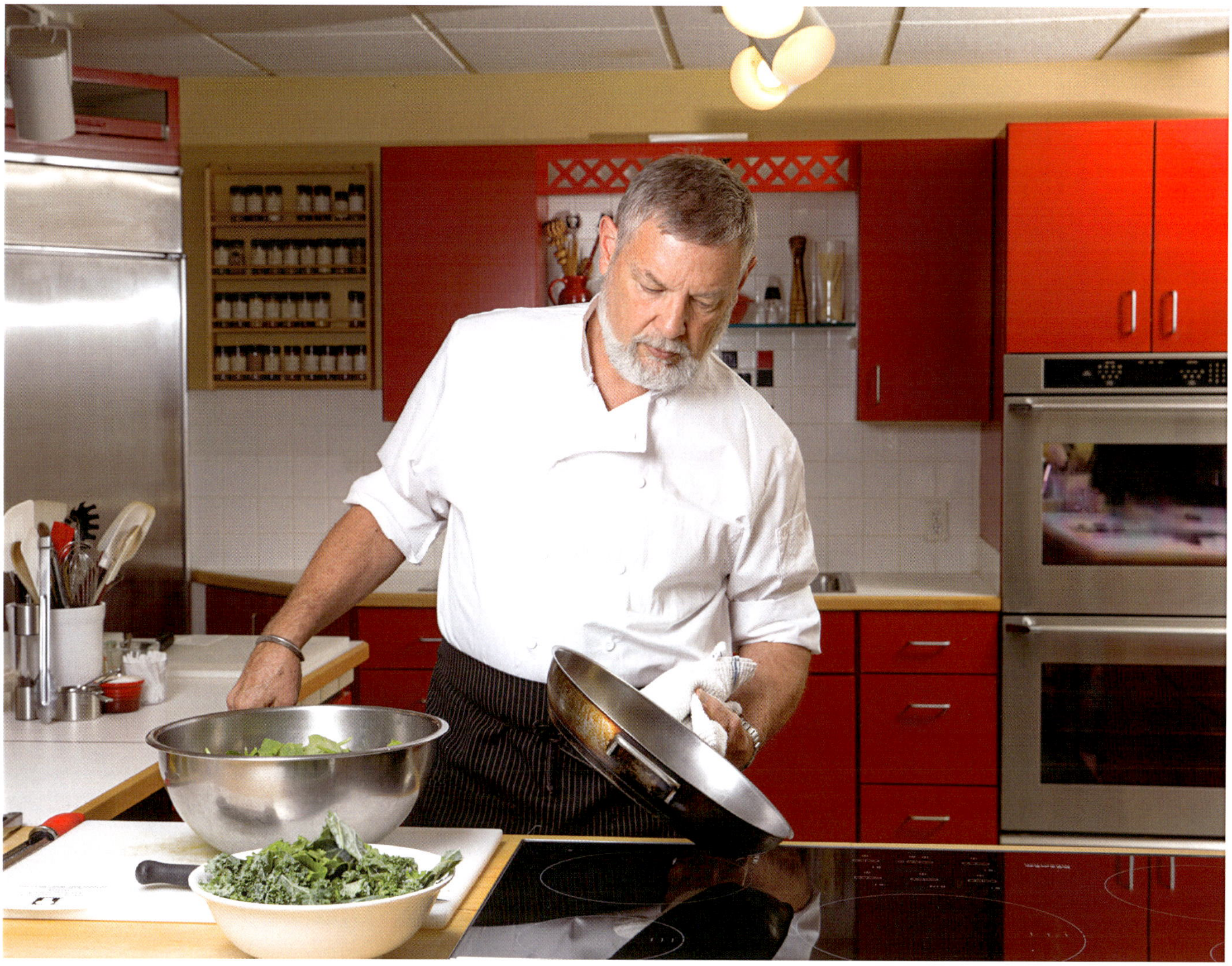

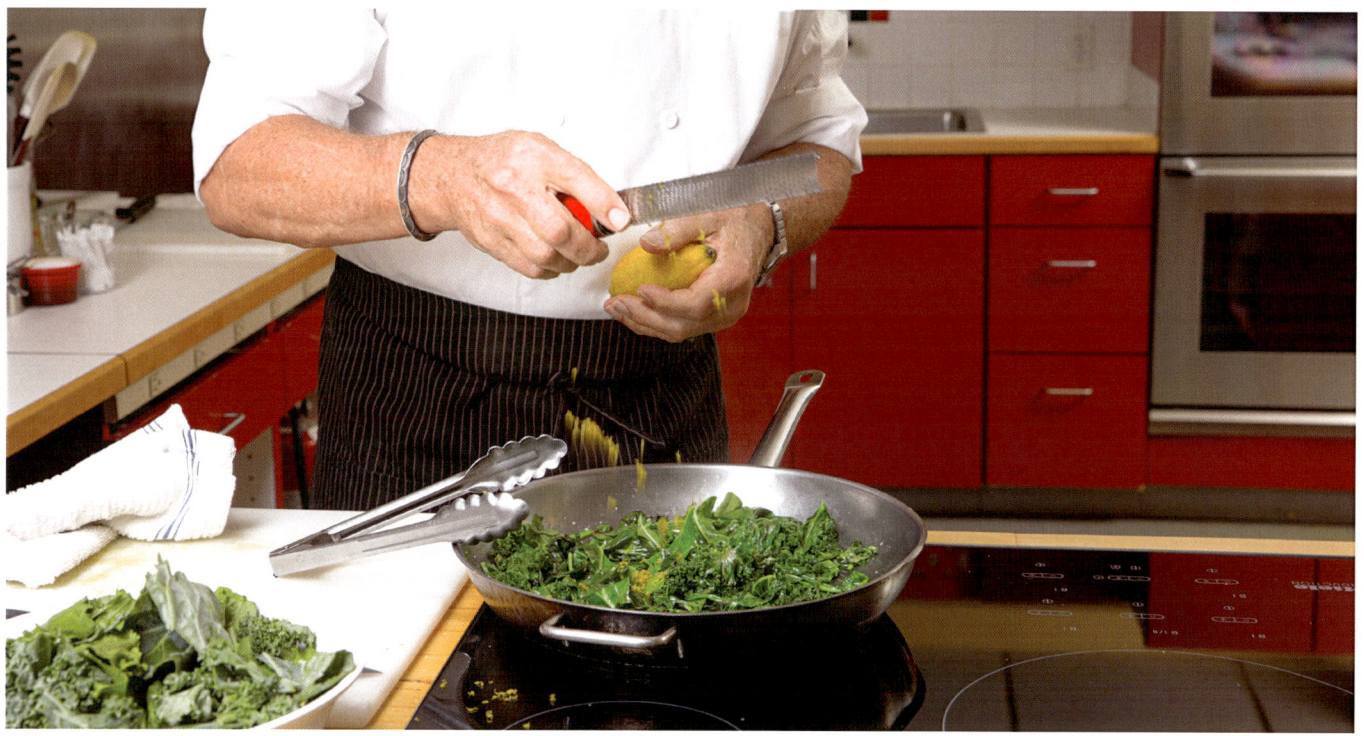

ROASTED PORK LOIN WITH MAPLE MUSTARD

Pork loin is an excellent cut of pork, as it is very affordable, and always comes out tender and juicy – if you remember to cook it to just medium! Anything more than medium results in a drier and tougher roast. The maple mustard glaze is a simple addition, and imparts a sweet and savory touch. Tamarind is a lovely fruit used in the Asian sub-continent, which has a tangy fruity flavor – similar to a dried apricot, but with an intriguing touch of sourness. It is found in a paste or a concentrate, and it is well worth making the trip to your local Asian market to purchase a jar. It has a long shelf life.

Make Hot and Fresh	**Serve The Next Day Cold**
Green Beans with Pecans, Baked Sweet Potatoes	Orange Tamarind Vinaigrette
Makes 4 Servings	*Makes 1 Serving*

Baked Sweet Potatoes

4 each small sweet potatoes, any variety

1 Tbsp olive oil
Salt and pepper

Preheat oven to 375°F.

Scrub the potatoes, then prick a few times with a fork and rub the skins with the olive oil. Season the skin with salt and pepper, place the potatoes on a baking sheet and bake on the middle rack of the oven for about 35-45 minutes, or until the potatoes are easily pierced with a skewer. Remove and keep warm.

Green Beans with Pecans

1 lb green beans, trimmed and halved on the diagonal

2 Tbsp olive oil
½ cup roasted and salted pecans, chopped

Salt and pepper

Bring a large pot of water to a full boil. Salt the water, add the beans, and cook until crisp tender, about 4 or 5 minutes. Drain, transfer immediately to a bowl of ice water, and let cool for 1 minute.

To serve hot, heat a skillet on medium heat. When hot, add the oil, pecans and beans and toss to coat. Add salt and pepper and cook, tossing and stirring occasionally, until the beans are heated through. Serve immediately.

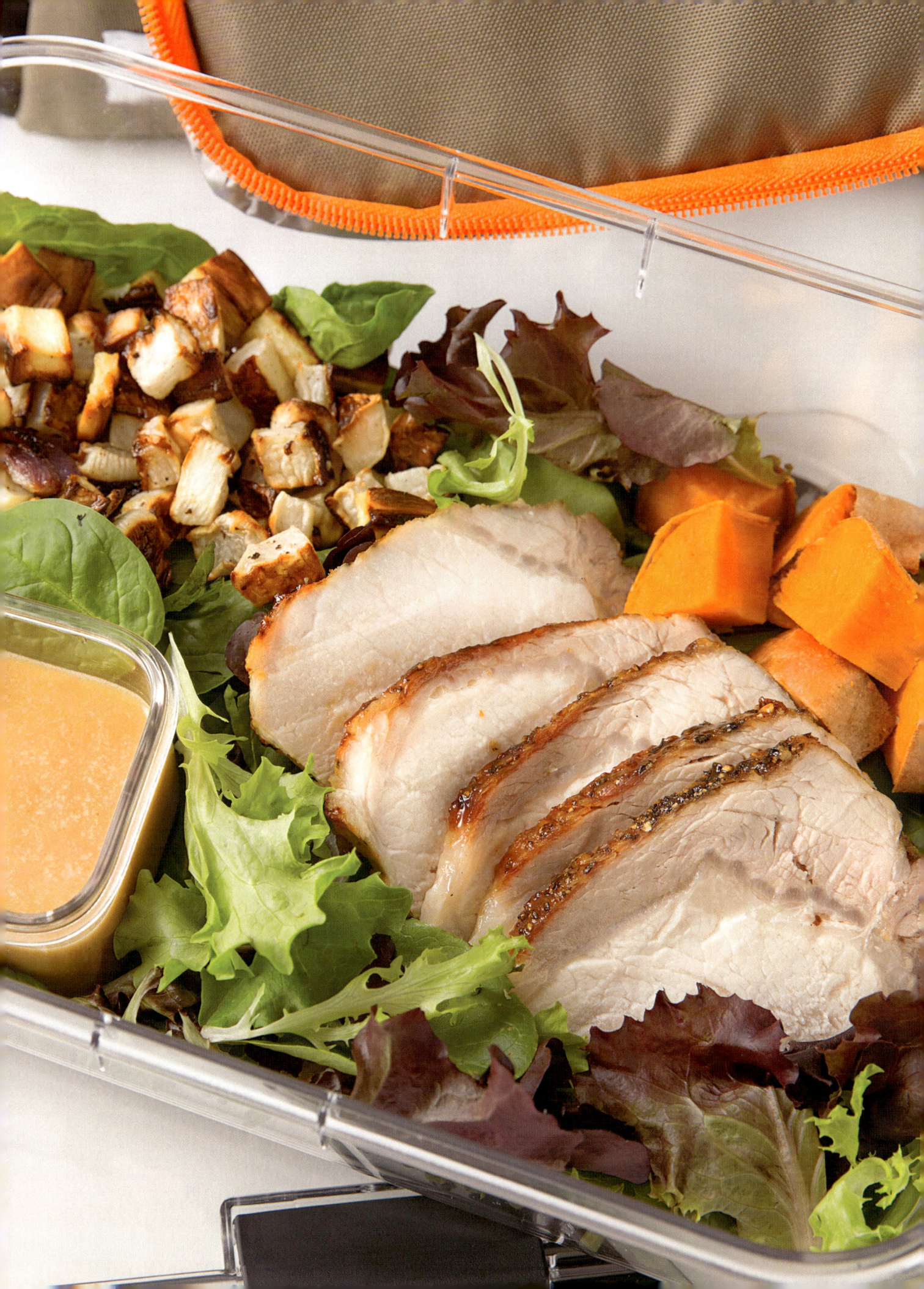

Roasted Pork Loin with Maple Mustard

¼ cup Dijon mustard
2 Tbsp maple syrup
1½ lbs pork loin
Salt and pepper
1 Tbsp grapeseed oil

Preheat oven to 375°F.

Mix the Dijon mustard and maple syrup together in a small mixing bowl. Set aside.

Heat a large skillet on high heat. Season the pork with salt and pepper. When the skillet is hot, add the oil and lay in the pork. Cook for 2 minutes on each side until lightly browned.

Place in the oven and roast for 20 minutes. Brush with some of the Maple Mustard and cook for another 10-20 minutes, depending on the thickness of the pork. Pork is cooked when it reaches an internal temperature of 140°F, or is very firm to the touch. When done, remove from the oven and let the pork rest for 5 minutes. Slice thin and serve with the remaining Maple Mustard.

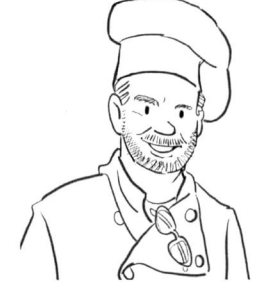

Trichinosis is no longer a concern in the United States. There is no need to cook your pork to medium well.

SERVE THE NEXT DAY COLD
Orange Tamarind Vinaigrette

Orange Tamarind Vinaigrette

2 cups fresh, no-pulp orange juice or ⅓ cup concentrate

1 lime, juiced
1 Tbsp rice wine vinegar
1 Tbsp tamarind paste
1 Tbsp raw honey
Salt
Tabasco, to taste
½ to ⅔ cup grape seed oil

½ red bell pepper, stemmed, seeded and minced

If using fresh orange juice, place in a medium sauce pot and bring to a boil. Reduce the juice until it starts to thicken and begins to darken in color, about 5-7 minutes. Remove, transfer to a large mixing bowl, and let cool.

Mix the orange juice reduction or the concentrate, lime juice, vinegar, tamarind, honey, salt and Tabasco. While whisking, slowly add ½ cup of oil. Add more oil, if needed, until the flavors are balanced. Taste and adjust the salt, Tabasco and honey. Stir in the red bell pepper. Makes about 1 cup

To Assemble

Large handful mixed greens

1 small Baked Sweet Potato, cut in ½-inch cubes

½ cup Green Beans with Pecans

5-6 oz Roasted Pork Loin, sliced thin

¼ cup Orange Tamarind Vinaigrette

Place the greens in one travel container; potato, the green beans and the pork loin in a second container; and the vinaigrette in a third. When ready to eat, toss all ingredients together.

SPICE RUBBED PORK TENDERLOIN

Although I generally do not preach measuring out items precisely, since we are using a rub here it is beneficial to actually measure out the salt in combination with the other seasonings. Amaranth is an under-appreciated seed, which is very easy to cook. Gluten-free and highly nutritious, it can be used anywhere that rice is used in your basic cooking. It is a great grain alternative, packed with protein, and with a wonderfully earthy nutty flavor. I love fruit based sauces and salsas for chicken, fish and pork, which are all complemented by the sweetness of the fruit. Careful with the snow peas, they cook very quickly and come both with and without the calyx or fibrous string that is common to many peas and beans.

Make Hot and Fresh
Amaranth, Mango Vinaigrette,
Lightly Steamed Snow Peas
Makes 4 Servings

Serve The Next Day Cold
Lettuce Wraps
Makes 1 Serving

Amaranth

1 cup amaranth
3 cups chicken stock
Salt and pepper

Place all ingredients in a medium saucepot. Stir once and bring to a boil. Reduce to a simmer and cover. Cook for 20-25 minutes or until amaranth is tender and all liquid is absorbed.

Keep covered until ready to serve or uncover, let cool, and reheat when ready to eat. Makes about 2 cups

Mango Vinaigrette

1 mango, peeled, pulp cut
  from seed
3 Tbsp rice vinegar
2 Tbsp lime juice
1 Tbsp raw honey
1 Tbsp mild chili powder
Salt
½ cup avocado oil

Purée mango, rice vinegar, lime juice, honey, chili powder and salt in food processor. With the motor running, slowly add the oil. Taste and adjust the seasonings. Place in a bowl, cover and refrigerate until ready to serve. Makes about 1½ cups

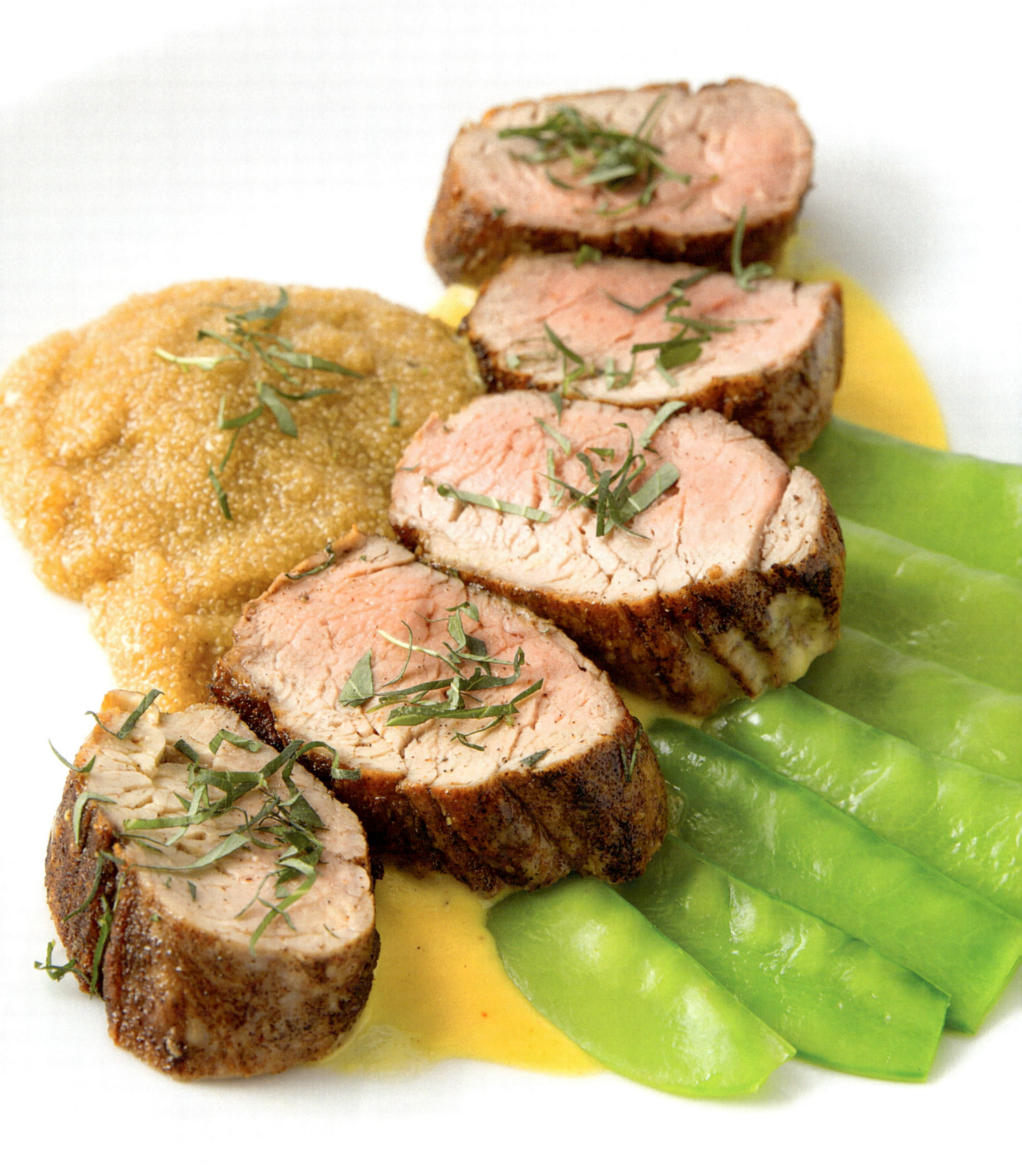

Lightly Steamed Snow Peas

8 oz snow peas, calyx (fibrous string) removed

Place 2 inches of water in a medium sauce pot. Set in a steamer basket and cover. Bring to a boil. Remove lid and add snow peas to the steamer basket. Cover and cook for only 20-25 seconds. Remove and serve immediately.

If not serving right away, place snow peas in a bowl of ice water to halt the cooking process. Drain and serve cold or reheat in the steamer for 10-15 seconds.

Spice Rubbed Pork Tenderloin

½ Tbsp salt
1 tsp ground allspice
Pinch cayenne
2 pork tenderloins, about 12-16 oz each
1 Tbsp avocado oil

Preheat oven to 375°F.

Stir together the salt, allspice, and cayenne. Pat the pork dry and sprinkle the spice rub all over pork, pressing to adhere.

Heat a large skillet over medium high heat. When hot, add the oil and heat until hot, but not smoking. Brown the pork tenderloins for about 1-2 minutes on all sides. Place the skillet in the middle of the oven for about 18-22 minutes, or until a digital read thermometer inserted into the center of each tenderloin registers 140°F. Remove and let the pork stand for about 5 minutes prior to serving. Slice thin.

SERVE THE NEXT DAY COLD
Lettuce Wraps

To Assemble

¼ cup Mango Vinaigrette
4 oz Spice Rubbed Pork Tenderloin
⅓ cup Amaranth
⅓ cup Steamed Snow Peas
4 large Bibb lettuce leaves, washed and dried

Pack each item separately in its own travel container. When ready to eat, place small portions of each item onto the lettuce leaves, wrap and serve.

GRILLED PORK CHOPS

Tapenade is a classic Mediterranean condiment boasting a tangy bright taste, and a briny flavor heavy with garlic and lemon. There are a wide variety of tapenades and they are easily found in natural food and ethnic markets. Legumes, like the lentils here, have been part of civilized food for ages, and are a great vehicle for other flavors. They are relatively simple to cook and are a good source of fiber and nutrition. I am noticing them more and more on bistro menus across town, packed with different flavorings, which is encouraging to see.

Make Hot and Fresh	**Serve The Next Day Cold**
Green Olive Tapenade, Green Lentils,	Bed of Mixed Greens
Steamed Carrots	with Citrus Vinaigrette
Makes 4 Servings	*Makes 1 Serving*

Green Olive Tapenade

1 cup Sicilian or Greek green olives, pitted

2 cloves garlic, peeled
Optional, 1 anchovy
1 Tbsp lemon juice, or to taste

2 Tbsp stemmed fresh oregano

¼ cup olive oil
Salt and pepper

In a food processor, add the olives, garlic, anchovy, lemon juice and oregano and pulse until roughly chopped. Transfer to a mixing bowl and add the olive oil. Season with salt and pepper, taste and adjust the seasonings, adding more lemon juice if needed, and set aside. Makes about 1 cup

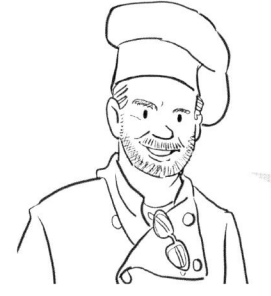

When serving firm, fibrous raw vegetables, they are much more enjoyable to the bite when they are sliced very thin. Consider buying a kitchen mandolin and safety glove, available at any cook store in multiple price points.

Green Lentils

1 cup green lentils
Salt
1 Tbsp olive oil

Rinse the lentils in a strainer under cold running water. Place the lentils in a small sauce pot and add enough cold water to cover them by about 1 inch. Bring to a boil and add salt. Reduce to a simmer and cook for about 16-20 minutes, until the lentils are tender to the bite. Remove and drain. Toss with the olive oil and a pinch of salt, cover and keep warm until ready to serve.

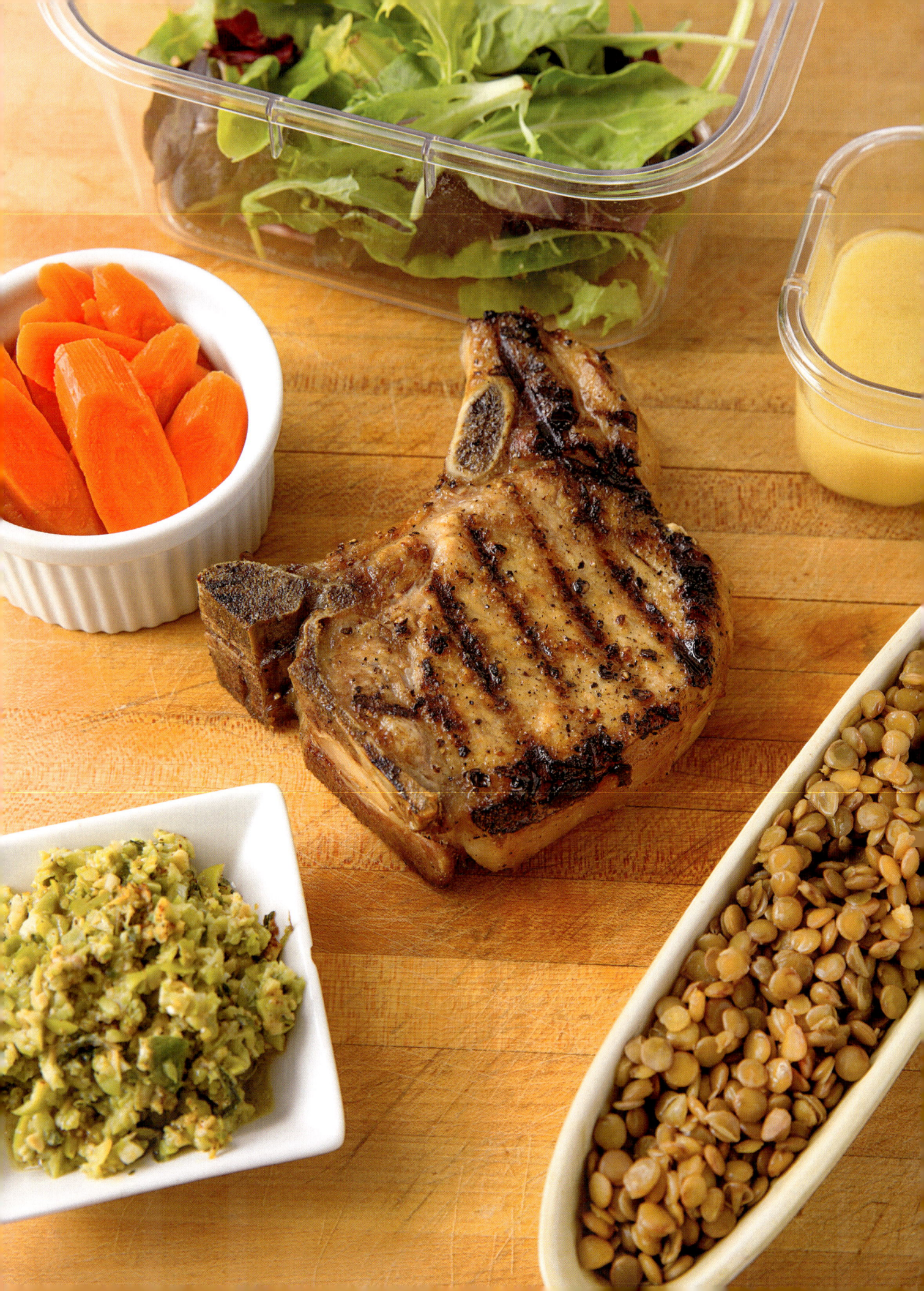

Steamed Carrots

1 lb carrots, scrubbed and sliced ⅛ inch thick	Place 2 inches of water in a medium sauce pot. Set in a steamer basket and cover. Bring to a boil. Remove lid and add the carrots to the steamer basket. Cover and cook for 3-4 minutes. Remove and serve immediately, or place the carrots in a bowl of ice water to halt the cooking process. Drain and serve cold, or reheat in the steamer for 30 seconds.

Grilled Pork Chops

4 each 6-8 oz boneless pork chops, about 1-inch thick	Heat a grill or cast iron skillet on medium high heat.
Salt and pepper	Season the chops generously with salt and pepper, patting the seasonings into the meat. Brush both sides with olive oil. Place the chops on the grill or skillet and cook for 6-8 minutes. Turn the chops over and cook for an additional 6-8 minutes, or until the chops are firm to the touch. Pork should be cooked to medium. Remove and serve.
1 Tbsp olive oil	

SERVE THE NEXT DAY COLD
Mixed Greens with Citrus Vinaigrette

Citrus Vinaigrette

1 shallot, minced	In the bottom of a salad bowl, combine the shallot, Dijon mustard, lemon juice, vinegar, salt and pepper and mix well with a fork or wire whip. While whisking, slowly add the olive oil in a thin stream. Properly done, the dressing will emulsify and not separate. Taste and adjust seasonings, if necessary.
2 Tbsp Dijon mustard	
2 Tbsp lemon juice	
2 Tbsp rice vinegar	
Salt and pepper	
⅔ cup extra-virgin olive oil	

To Assemble

Large handful mixed greens	Place the greens in one travel container; the chops, lentils and carrots in a second container; and the vinaigrette in a third. If adding the tapenade, place in a fourth container. When ready to eat, toss all ingredients together in a bowl and serve.
¼ cup Citrus Vinaigrette	
5 oz Grilled Pork Chops, sliced thin	
⅓ cup Green Lentils	
⅓ cup Steamed Carrots	
Optional, 2 Tbsp Green Olive Tapenade	

ITALIAN SAUSAGE, BRAISED FENNEL, PEPPERS AND ROMA TOMATOES

This is Italian comfort food – homey, down-to-earth and rich, and as welcoming as a big hug! Sausage and peppers are a traditional pairing, and the addition of fresh tomatoes and fennel adds another level of flavor and texture, and creates a delicious stew that pairs perfectly with creamy grits. These hominy grits are simple and highly nutritious, and although generally served as a breakfast dish, I like them at any time of the day.

Make Hot and Fresh
Braised Fennel, Peppers, Roma Tomatoes, Hominy Grits
Makes 4 Servings

Serve the Next Day Hot
Makes 1 Serving

Italian Sausage, Braised Fennel, Peppers and Roma Tomatoes

1½ lbs fresh Italian sausage, sweet or spicy

1 large fennel bulb
4 medium tomatoes
2 Tbsp olive oil
1 large onion, sliced thin
2 red bell peppers, sliced thin

Salt and pepper
2-3 cloves garlic, minced
Optional, ½ cup dry red wine

2 Tbsp stemmed and minced Italian parsley

1 Tbsp stemmed and minced fresh oregano

Optional, 2-3 Tbsp grated fresh Parmesan cheese

Preheat oven to 375°F.

Place the sausage on a metal sheet pan and place in the oven. Cook until very springy to the touch, about 12-15 minutes. Remove and keep warm.

Rinse the fennel bulb and cut off the tall stalks at the top of the bulb and discard. Split the fennel bulb in half from top to bottom and cut out the core. Slice the fennel bulb across the ribs into very thin strips, about $1/16$ -inch wide. Using a serrated vegetable peeler, peel, seed and juice the tomatoes, then chop them into rough chunks, about ½-inch in size.

Heat a large skillet on high heat. When hot, add the olive oil. When the oil is hot, add the onions, peppers and fennel. Season with salt and pepper. Reduce the heat to medium. Cook for 3-4 minutes, stirring occasionally, until the vegetables begin to soften. Add the garlic and cook for another few seconds. If using, add the red wine and increase the heat to high. Reduce the wine to almost evaporated, being careful not to scorch the wine. Immediately add the tomatoes.

Reduce the heat to a simmer and cook for about 10 minutes, or until the mixture starts to thicken. Stir in the herbs and taste and adjust the seasonings.

Slice the sausage into ¼-inch thick slices, cutting slightly on the bias, and add the sausages to the vegetable mixture. Keep warm until ready to serve. Serve on top of the grits. Garnish with Parmesan cheese.

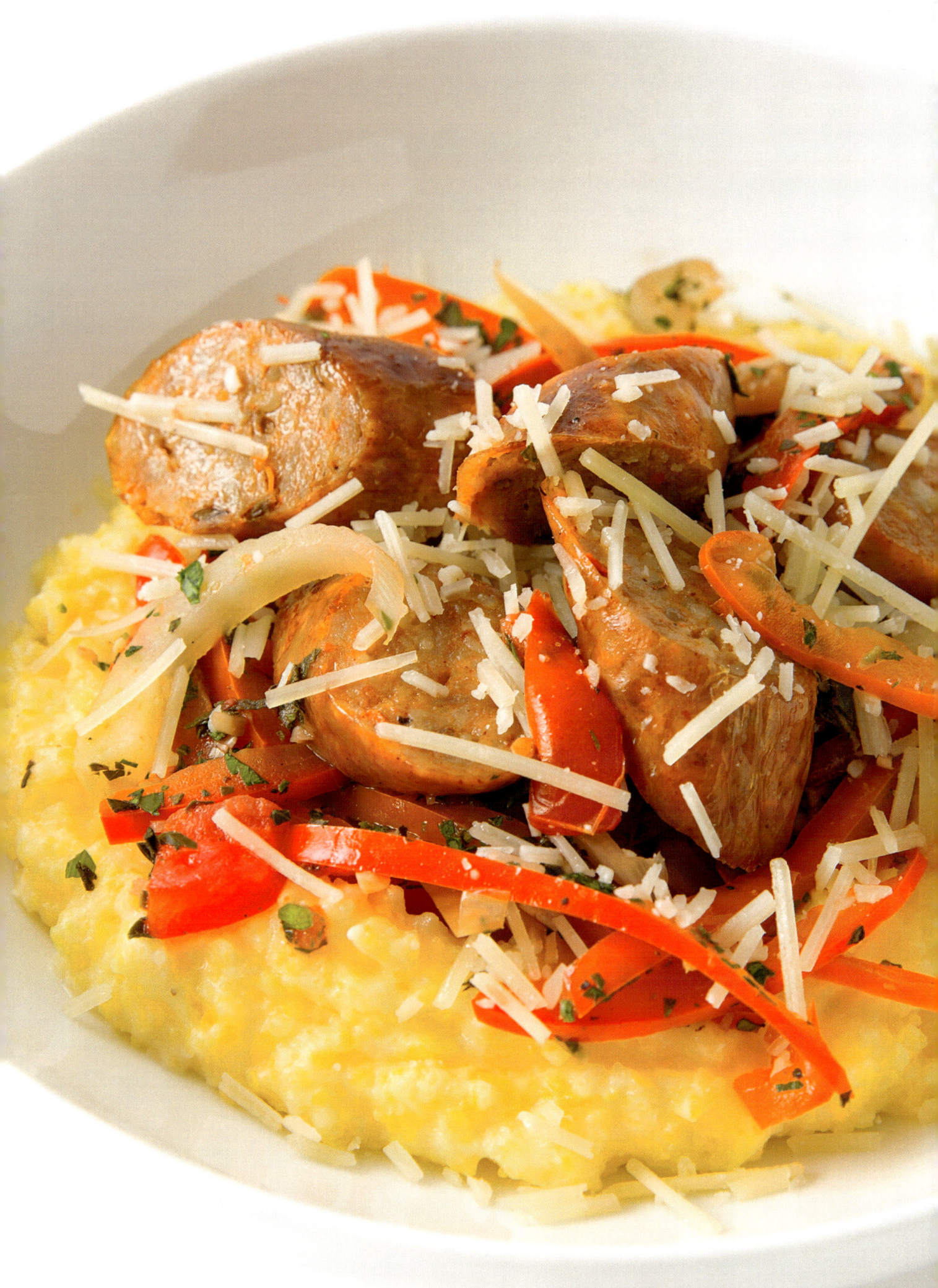

Hominy Grits

4 cups water
1 Tbsp salt
1 cup hominy grits
Optional, ⅓ cup grated
  Parmesan cheese

2 Tbsp unsalted butter

In a large saucepot, add water and salt and bring to a boil. Add the grits to the water in a thin steady stream, while stirring continuously with a high temperature rubber spatula or wooden spoon. When all the grits have been added, reduce the heat to a simmer.

Continue cooking for approximately 10-15 minutes, stirring often, until the grits are cooked, soft and creamy to the bite. The grits will begin pulling away from the sides of the pot when they are almost done. Remove the pot from the heat and add the cheese and butter. This is the basic technique for cooking all grits. Makes about 4 cups

NOTE: Grits can be spread on a greased or parchment lined sheet pan, cooled, covered and refrigerated, then cut and reheated in an oven or microwave.

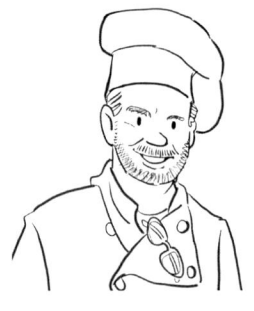

For dishes such as this Italian Sausage with Braised Fennel, Peppers and Roma Tomatoes that are to be served hot the next day, the quantities are totally up to you, and depend upon your appetite!

SERVE THE NEXT DAY HOT

½ cup Hominy Grits
1½ - 2 cups Italian
  Sausage with Fennel,
  Peppers and Tomatoes

Optional, 2 Tbsp, grated
  Parmesan cheese

Place grits in a microwave-proof travel container, add Italian Sausage mixture and cheese, if desired. When ready to eat, sprinkle 1 Tbsp water on top, loosely place the lid on and reheat for 3-4 minutes.

PORK ARRACHERAS

You can use any thinly sliced meat found in your market or butcher shop to make Arracheras. They only take a few minutes to cook on a hot surface. You don't have to marinate them but it does add to the flavor. Sweet potato pancakes are as easy to make as any pancake and they reheat beautifully. This salsa is vibrant in color and offers a delicious balance of sweetness and heat. Many thanks to my good friend Cathy Harokopis for inspiring me on this and many modern Mexican cuisine ideas!

Make Hot and Fresh
Sweet Potato Pancakes, Grilled Jalapeño Orange Salsa, Crunchy Slaw
Makes 4 Servings

Serve The Next Day Cold
Makes 1 Serving

Sweet Potato Pancakes

3 eggs
1 Tbsp arrowroot
Salt and pepper
2 cups sweet potato, shredded
Avocado oil for frying

In a medium sized bowl, beat the eggs with the arrowroot, salt and pepper. Mix in the sweet potatoes until well combined.

Heat a large frying pan over medium-high heat, then add enough oil to lightly coat the bottom of the pan. Drop spoonfuls of the mixture into the pan, about 3 inches round, and cook for 3 minutes on each side until golden brown, flipping only once.

Crunchy Slaw

4 cups shredded green cabbage

8 large radishes, trimmed and julienned

3 green onions, trimmed and sliced thin

¼ cup chopped cilantro
2 Tbsp lime juice
2 Tbsp olive oil
Salt and pepper
1 Tbsp raw honey

Mix everything in a large bowl. Cover and refrigerate until ready to serve. Makes about 4 cups

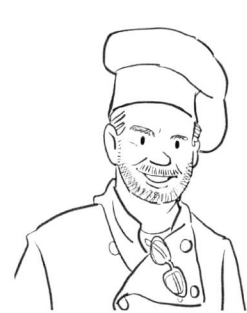

As well as being a valuable emulsifier, and a welcome accompaniment to different meats and cold cuts, any mustard is a versatile condiment that adds flavor and texture to any sauce, glaze, dressing or marinade.
Have fun and experiment!

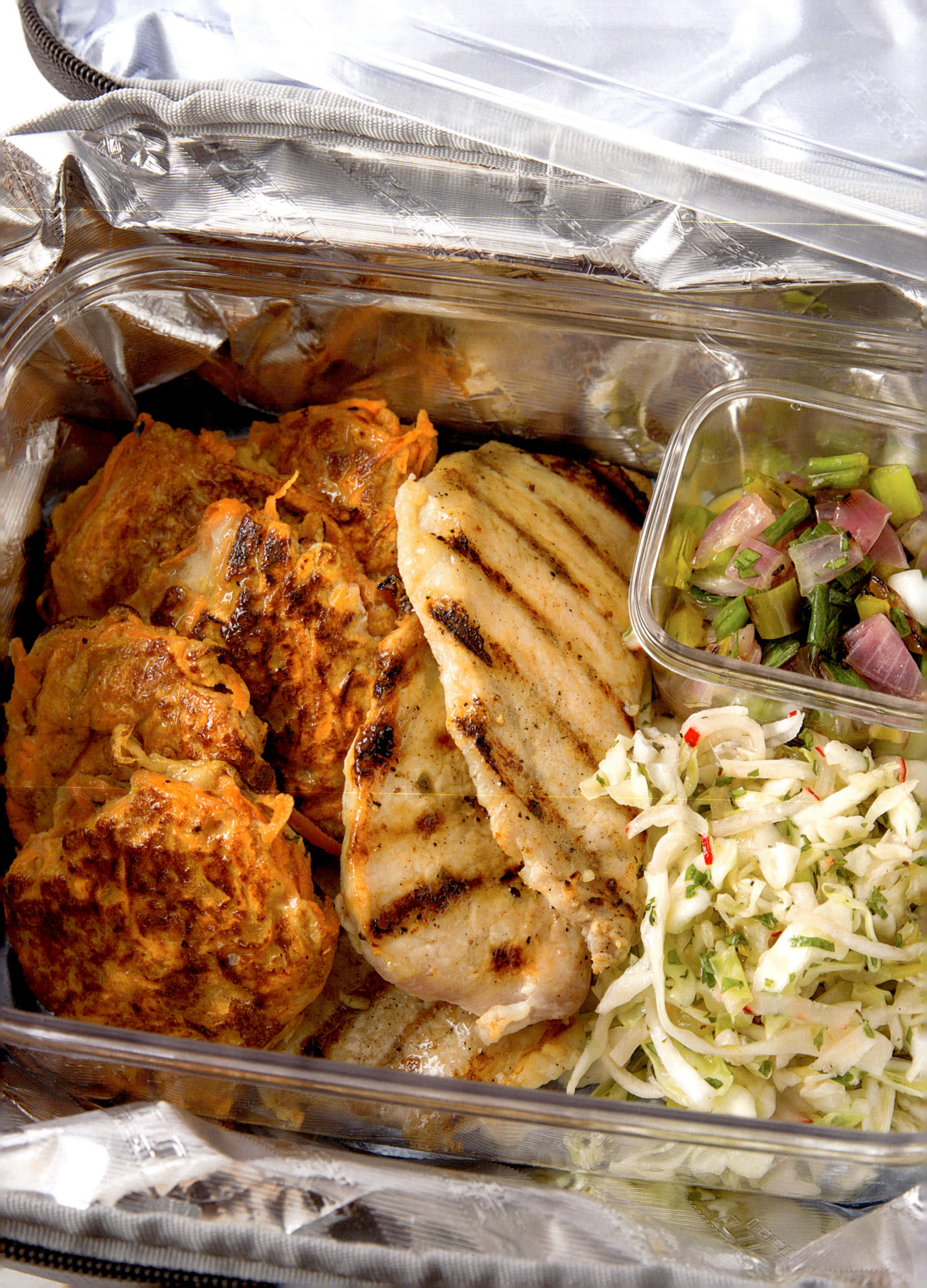

Grilled Jalapeño Orange Salsa

1 small red onion, cut
   into ½-inch thick slices

1 jalapeño, stemmed,
   split and seeded

1 Tbsp olive oil
8 green onions, trimmed
   to 6 inches
½ cup orange juice
2 Tbsp lime juice
3 Tbsp chopped cilantro
Salt

Heat a grill or cast iron skillet on high heat.

Lightly oil the red onion and jalapeño. Lay on the grill or skillet and cook for about 3 minutes per side, or until the pepper is browned on all sides and the onions are lightly charred. Remove and place in a food processor. Grill the green onions for about 20 seconds per side and add to food processor. Add the juices, cilantro and salt and pulse chop until your desired consistency. Makes about 1½ cups

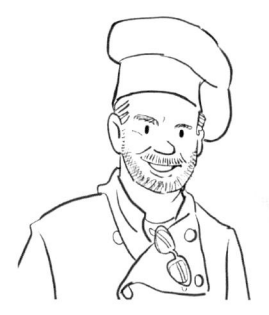

Try this salsa with different chiles – the jalapeños which I have used here offer a medium level of spice, but for extra kick, opt for a habanero instead, which will add some serious heat to your meal!

Pork Arracheras

2 jalapeños, stemmed,
   seeded and minced

2 Tbsp olive oil
2 Tbsp lime juice
4 garlic cloves, minced
Salt and pepper
1½ lbs thinly cut
   boneless pork chops

In a mixing bowl, combine the jalapeños, oil, lime juice, garlic, salt and pepper. Coat the pork with the marinade, cover and refrigerate for 30 minutes or up to 2 hours.

Heat a grill or cast iron skillet on high heat. Scrape off the excess marinade. Cook the pork for about 3-4 minutes, then turn over and cook for an additional 3-5 minutes, or until firm to the touch. Remove and serve.

SERVE THE NEXT DAY COLD

To Assemble

2 Sweet Potato Pancakes
⅔ cup Crunchy Slaw
5 oz Pork Arracheras
¼ cup Grilled Jalapeño
   Orange Salsa

Pack each item separately. To serve, top the pancakes with the slaw, then the pork, and drizzle with salsa.

GRILLED LAMB CHOPS

This is a great summer dish. Lamb is generally more expensive than other meats, and is also tricky to re-heat successfully, so these lamb chops are the only market available cut I like to use when thinking about using them for make-and-take meals. Grilling the romaine creates an amazing flavor transformation and offers an unusual take on an everyday salad. By making the New Potato Salad with a vinaigrette, instead of mayonnaise, we are making an American mainstay a healthier food choice. The Walnut Pesto is a simple healthy garnish that complements many of the dishes in this book.

Serve Hot and Fresh	**Serve The Next Day Cold**
New Potato Salad, Grilled Hearts of Romaine, Walnut Pesto	*Makes 1 Serving*
Makes 4 Servings	

New Potato Salad

1½ lbs new potatoes or fingerling potatoes, scrubbed

Salt and pepper
1 shallot, minced
1 Tbsp Dijon mustard
3 Tbsp sherry vinegar
½ cup olive oil
6 oz Black Forest ham
2 Tbsp minced fresh Italian parsley

Rinse the potatoes under cold water and place in a medium saucepot. Add a large pinch of salt and cover the potatoes with cold water. Bring to a boil and reduce to a simmer. Cook for 10-20 minutes, depending upon the size of the potatoes, or until you can prick them with a wooden skewer or toothpick and they are tender. Drain and let cool, then cut in ¼-inch thick rounds.

In a large salad bowl, whisk together the shallot, mustard and vinegar. Whisking constantly, gradually pour in the olive oil to form an emulsion. Season well with salt and pepper.

Add the potatoes, ham and parsley to the vinaigrette. Toss gently to coat, taste and adjust seasonings. Cover and refrigerate until ready to use. Makes about 1 quart

Walnut Pesto

½ cup walnut halves
2 cloves garlic
1 Tbsp cold water
½ cup walnut oil
Salt and pepper
1 Tbsp chopped Italian parsley

In a small food processor, grind the walnuts and the garlic until well ground. With the motor running, add the water and the oil to make a smooth paste. Transfer to a small mixing bowl and add the salt, pepper and parsley. Cover and set aside.

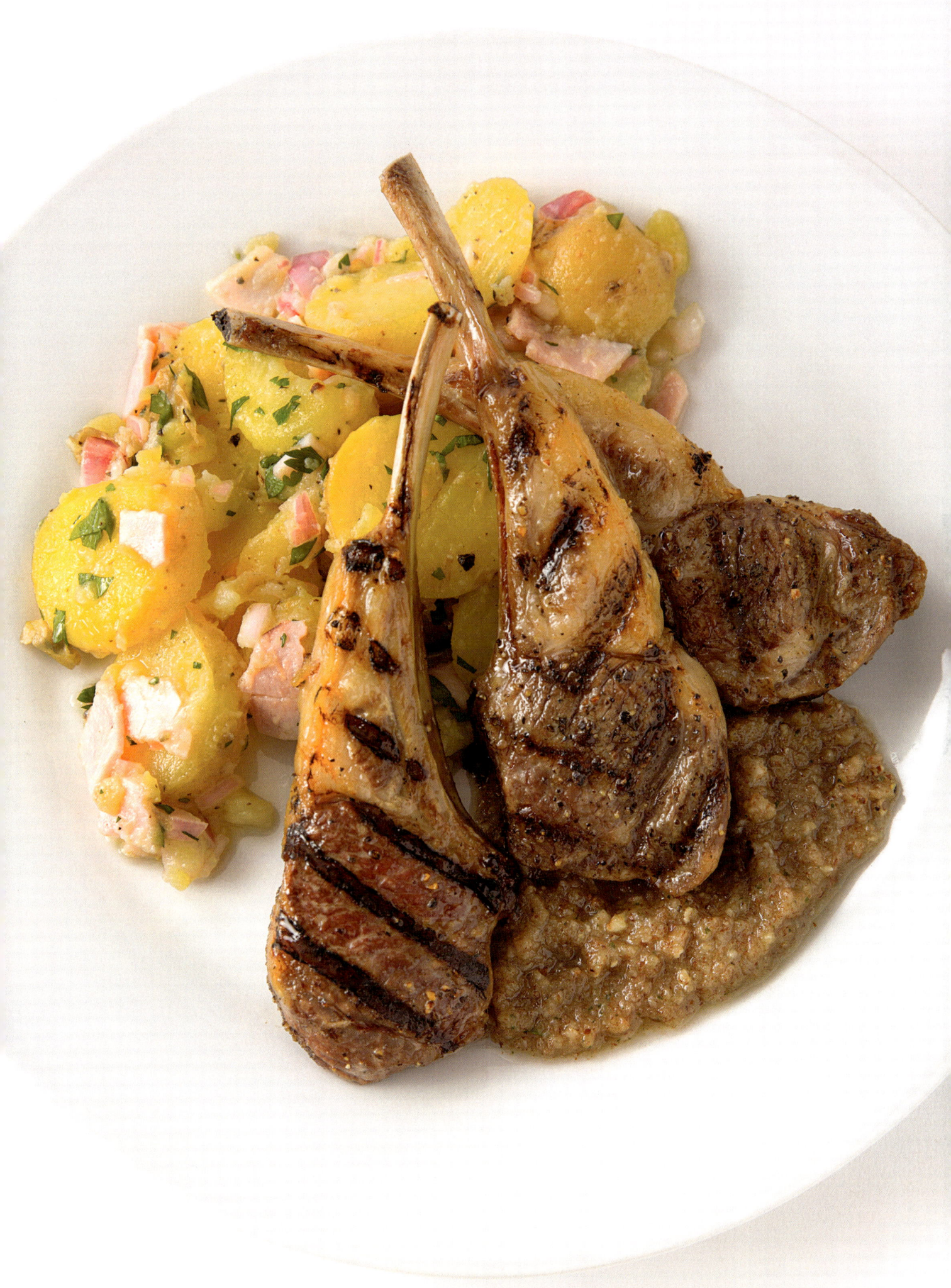

Grilled Lamb Chops

12 lamb chops, rib or loin chops

Salt and pepper
Olive oil

Heat a grill or cast iron skillet on medium high heat.

Season the chops with salt and pepper and brush with olive oil. When the grill or skillet is hot, add the lamb chops. Cook for 5-6 minutes, then turn over and cook for an additional 5-6 minutes. At this point, the chops are rare. Add 1-2 more minutes per degree of desired doneness. I enjoy mine at medium rare. Remove and set aside to cool slightly.

Grilled Hearts of Romaine

Olive oil
2 hearts of romaine
2 Tbsp olive oil
Salt and pepper

Heat a grill or cast iron skillet on high heat.

If necessary, wash and trim the romaine and split in half lengthwise, keeping the core intact. This will hold the leaves together. Brush the cut side of the romaine with olive oil, then season with salt and pepper. Place on the grill or skillet and cook for about 30-45 seconds, lightly wilting the lettuce and making slight char marks. Remove and let cool.

To Assemble

Carefully remove the core from each romaine half. Place the halves onto each plate, then top with New Potato Salad and arrange the Grilled Lamb Chops, bone side up, around the salad and serve immediately.

SERVE THE NEXT DAY COLD

To Assemble

3 Grilled Lamb Chops, boned and sliced thin

1 half Grilled Heart of Romaine

⅔ cup New Potato Salad

2 Tbsp Walnut Pesto

Pack each item in a separate travel container. When ready to serve, place potato salad on romaine, and top with lamb and pesto.

Walnut Pesto, from the family of Sauce Aillade, is a classic French condiment that can be served at room temperature and offers an excellent alternative to the traditional cheese-laden pestos that we are used to. It can be a great accompaniment to meats, fish or roasted vegetables.

GRILLED SHRIMP BROCHETTES

Shrimp is the most popular seafood in the USA, and for good reason. They are easy to cook and take on flavor extremely well. Shrimp are readily available nowadays at the store already peeled and de-veined for your convenience, saving you that tedious step. Here, we have paired them with a bright pesto vinaigrette – using parsley instead of the traditional basil – and a slaw based on jicama, a juicy tuber with a nutty flavor and a satisfying crunch. The Fresh Roasted Corn completes the dish with a burst of color and flavor. I use fresh corn in a wide variety of dishes, from soups to entrées.

Make Hot and Fresh
Parsley Pesto Vinaigrette, Jicama Ensalata,
Fresh Roasted Corn
Makes 4 Servings

Serve The Next Day Cold
Mixed Baby Greens
Makes 1 Serving

Jicama Ensalata

½ medium jicama,
  julienned

3-4 Tbsp seasoned rice
  vinegar

Salt
Sugar, to taste
½ Tbsp chili powder

In a mixing bowl, toss the ingredients together and adjust seasonings. Set aside.

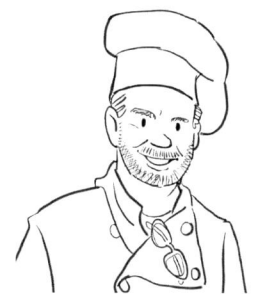

Grilling techniques don't change whether you are outdoors or indoors. The only difference is that grilling plates used indoors can make your kitchen smoky. Be prepared!

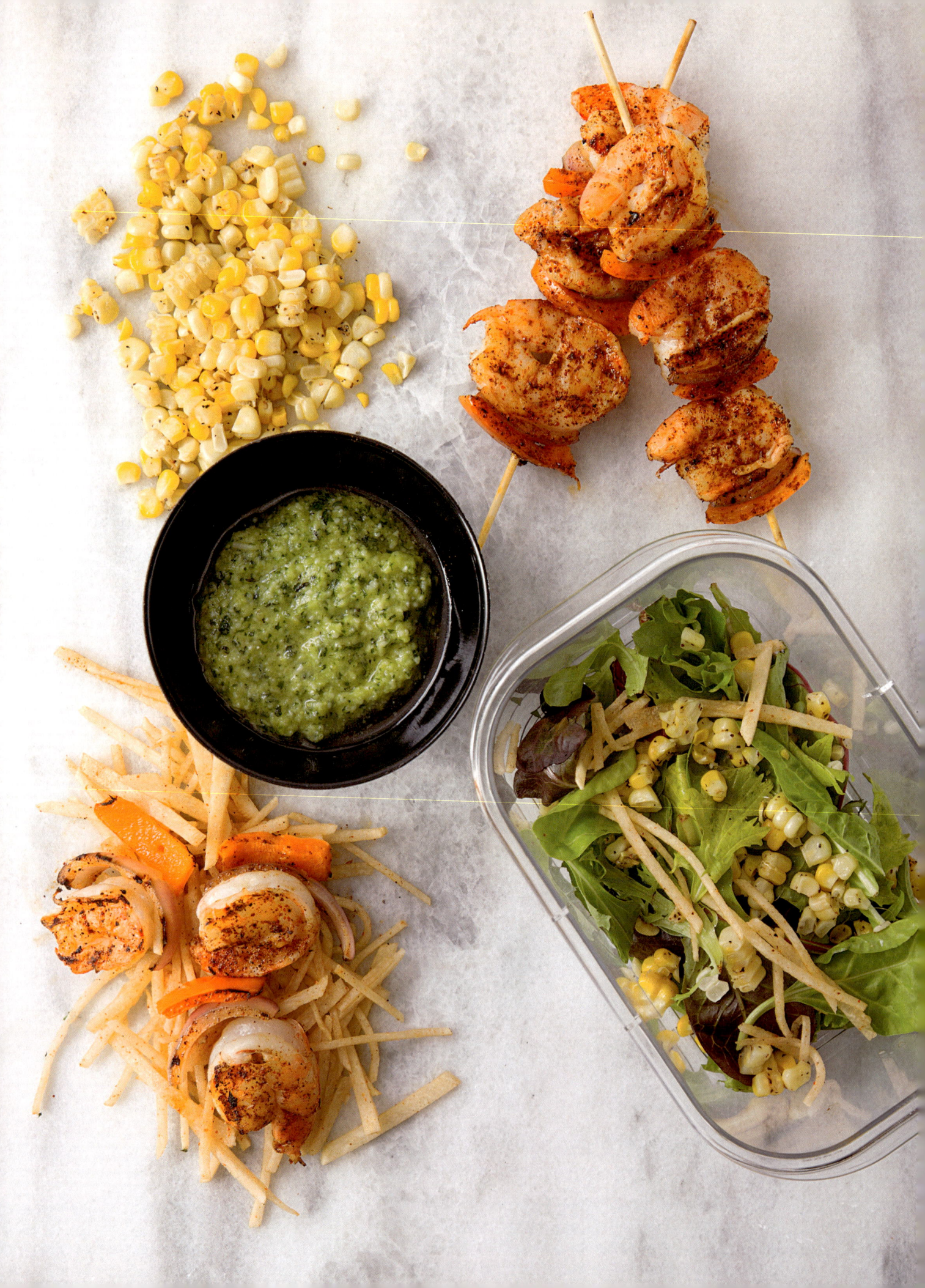

Parsley Pesto Vinaigrette

½ bunch Italian parsley, stemmed

2 Tbsp pine nuts

4 Tbsp grated Parmesan cheese

1 garlic clove, crushed

3 Tbsp white wine vinegar

1 Tbsp Dijon mustard

Salt and pepper

⅓ cup olive or avocado oil

Place parsley, pine nuts, Parmesan and garlic in a food processor and pulse to a coarse consistency.

In a medium mixing bowl, whisk the vinegar, mustard, salt and pepper together until dissolved. While continuing to whisk rapidly, add the oil slowly in a thin stream. Done properly, the dressing will emulsify. Stir in the pesto and taste and adjust seasonings.

The sauce will keep emulsified if refrigerated in a covered container for about 3 days. Makes about 1 cup

Fresh Roasted Corn

2 ears corn

1 Tbsp olive oil

Salt and pepper

Preheat oven to 400°F.

Shuck corn, remove all silk, rinse and pat dry. Oil the corn and season with salt and pepper. Wrap individually in aluminum foil and place in the center of the oven. Cook for 15-20 minutes. Remove and let cool. When cool, cut the corn from the cob.

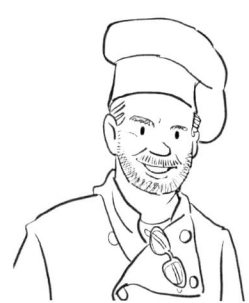

There are many different shapes into which vegetables can be cut — here the jicama is julienned, which is a matchstick cut, made up of short thin strips.

Grilled Shrimp Brochettes

Bamboo skewers
1 red bell pepper
3 Tbsp olive oil
Salt and pepper
1 small red onion
1¼ lbs large shrimp,
   peeled and deveined
1 Tbsp chili powder

If using bamboo skewers, soak in cold water for about 15 minutes.

Heat a grill or cast iron skillet on high heat.

Core and split the bell pepper and then press flat. Lightly brush both sides with olive oil and season. Place on grill, skin side down and cook for approximately 1 minute. Turn over and cook for an additional minute. Remove and let cool. The pepper should be a little undercooked. When cool, cut into ½-inch cubes.

Cut the onion into ½-inch slices, parallel to the equator of the onion. Season and brush both sides with olive oil and place on the grill, cut side down. Cook for approximately 2 minutes, then turn over and cook for another 2 minutes. Remove and let cool, then cut into ½-inch cubes.

NOTE: Make sure the peppers and onions are the same size as the shrimp —they must be the same width on the skewers. This helps them to cook evenly.

Using 4 each 8-inch or longer metal or bamboo skewers, thread the shrimp, onions and peppers alternately onto the skewers. Season with salt, pepper and chili powder, and then brush lightly with olive oil. Place on the grill and cook for approximately 2-3 minutes on each side, until the center of the shrimp is white and no longer pink.

Serve immediately, on top of the Jicama Ensalata and Fresh Roasted Corn and topped with Parsley Pesto Vinaigrette. Or, let shrimp cool to room temperature, then serve.

SERVE THE NEXT DAY COLD

To Assemble

2 oz mixed baby greens
1 Grilled Shrimp
   Brochette, skewer
   removed
¼ cup Fresh Roasted
   Corn
½ cup Jicama Ensalata
¼ cup Parsley Pesto
   Vinaigrette

Pack items in separate travel containers. When ready to eat, toss together all ingredients with the vinaigrette.

SHRIMP AND VEGETABLE STIR FRY

This cookbook wouldn't be complete without a nice classic stir fry. While there are a lot of curry pastes available in the markets, this particular curry is delicious and simple to make, plus you are sourcing your own ingredients. In addition, you are free to change up the vegetables and the proteins to your liking. Tamari is a gluten-free soy sauce. Chinese long beans can be found in Asian markets but green beans make an excellent substitute.

Make Hot and Fresh
Steamed Rice, Turmeric Ginger Curry,
Tamari
Makes 4 Servings

Serve The Next Day Hot
Makes 1 Serving

Steamed Rice

1 cup long grain white rice

2 cups water
Salt

Place all ingredients in a medium saucepot or rice cooker and stir once to moisten rice. Do not stir again during the entire cooking process. Place on high heat and bring to a boil. Cover the saucepot with a tight-fitting lid and reduce heat to low. Cook approximately 18-22 minutes or until all water is absorbed. Remove from heat and leave covered at least 5-10 minutes before serving. If using a rice cooker, use the white rice setting, which usually takes about 45 minutes. Makes about 3 cups

NOTE: There are a wide variety of white rices available in Asian markets. They vary in cooking time and rice to water ratio, so be careful to follow the package instruction on any new rice you try.

Turmeric Ginger Curry

1 Tbsp coconut oil
1 small onion, diced
1 clove garlic diced
2-inch fresh turmeric, peeled and grated, or 1 Tbsp ground

½ tsp cumin
2-inch ginger, diced
½ tsp fresh ground black pepper

Optional, 1 Tbsp Garam Masala

Heat a medium saucepot on medium heat. When hot, add the coconut oil, onion, garlic, turmeric, cumin, ginger, pepper and, if desired, garam masala. Sauté on a medium heat for 3-4 minutes, or until the onions become pale and translucent. Transfer to a small food processor and process to a rough paste. Set aside.

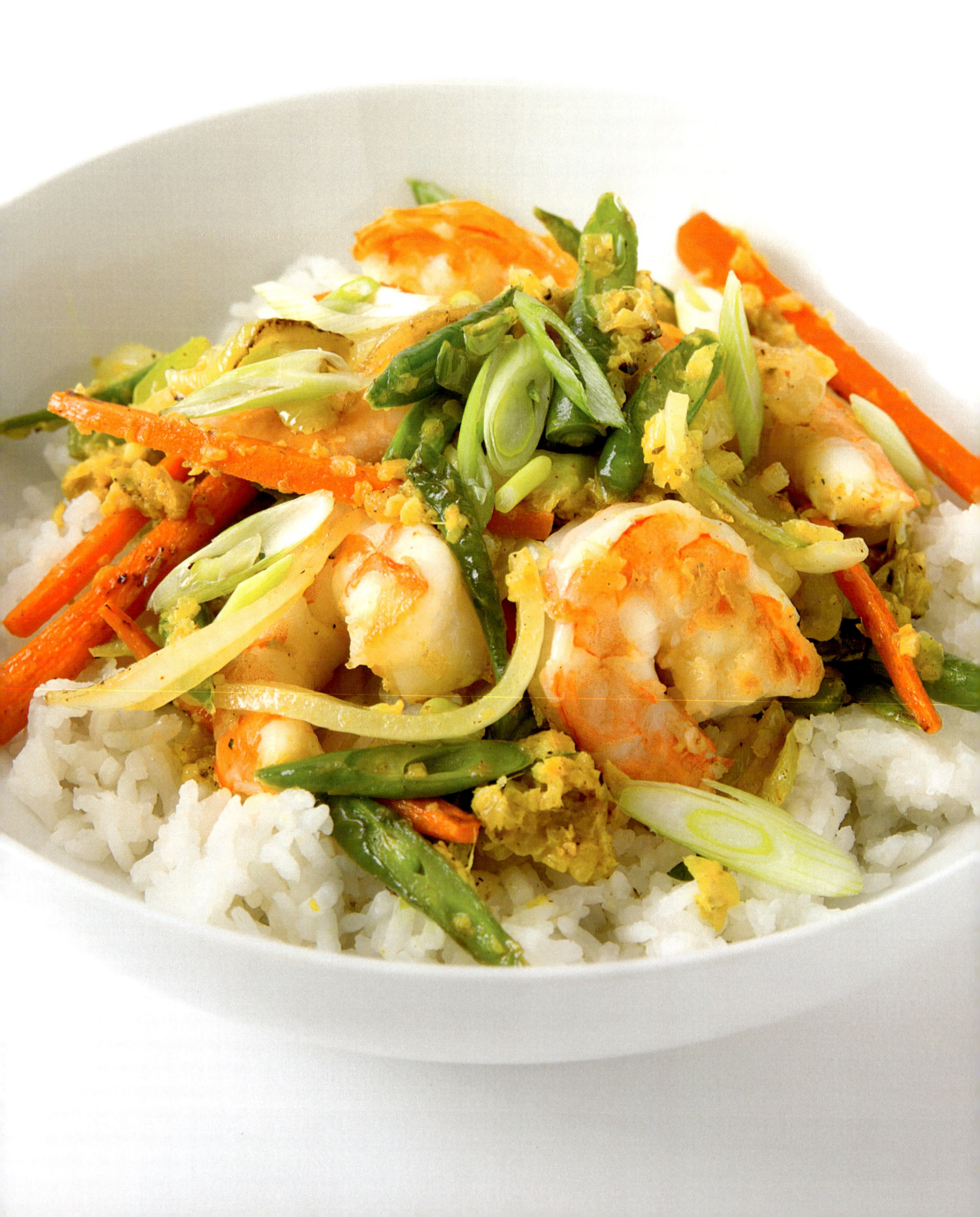

Shrimp and Vegetable Stir Fry

2 Tbsp olive oil, divided

2 Tbsp sesame oil, divided

24 oz medium shrimp, peeled and deveined

2 cloves garlic, minced

Pinch crushed red chili flakes

1 onion, julienned

1 carrot, peeled and julienned

1 head baby bok choy, trimmed and cut lengthwise in quarters

¼ lb Chinese long beans or green beans, trimmed and julienned

¼ cup Turmeric Ginger Curry

⅓ cup chicken stock

1 Tbsp Tamari

1 Tbsp arrowroot, dissolved in 1 Tbsp cold water

2 tsp sesame seeds

3 green onions, julienned

Heat a large wok or large skillet on high heat. When hot, add 1 Tbsp of each of the oils and the shrimp. Cook for about 2 minutes, stirring occasionally, until the shrimp are almost done. Remove and set aside. Return the pan to the stove and add more oil if needed. Add the garlic, and chili flakes and stir-fry just until they are aromatic, about 15 seconds. Remove the seasonings and set aside in a small dish.

Add the remaining oils to the wok. When hot, add the onion, carrots, bok choy and beans and stir-fry until the onions turn glossy and bright, about 2-3 minutes.

Add the Turmeric Ginger Curry, chicken stock and Tamari and bring to a boil. While stirring, add in the arrowroot slurry. Return the shrimp and seasonings to the pan and bring to boiling temperature. Serve immediately, garnished with sesame seeds and green onion.

SERVE THE NEXT DAY HOT

½ cup Steamed Rice

1½ cups Shrimp and Vegetable Stir Fry

Place the rice and stir fry in a microwave-proof travel container. When ready to serve, sprinkle with 1 Tbsp water, loosely cover and microwave for 3-4 minutes. Serve immediately.

GRILLED SALMON

Salmon is one of the only types of fish that eats well both hot and cold, and really does lend itself very successfully to a variety of cooking mediums. It goes very well with a wide variety of flavors. This Gazpacho Sauce, which is based on the soup of the same name, is bursting with flavor and nutrition. The recipe makes a lot but keeps for 3-4 days and can be served with a variety of proteins. You can also add tomato juice and, voilà! Summer Soup! The Quinoa Pilaf and Grilled Vegetables, once tasted for the first time, will become a mainstay in your everyday kitchen.

Make Hot and Fresh
Gazpacho Sauce, Quinoa Pilaf,
Grilled Vegetables
Makes 4 Servings

Serve the Next Day Cold
Shredded Romaine, Chili Lime Vinaigrette
Makes 1 Serving

Quinoa Pilaf

1 Tbsp olive oil
½ yellow onion, minced
1 stalk celery, washed
  and minced

1 small carrot, minced
½ tsp dry thyme
1 bay leaf
¾ cup quinoa, rinsed
1½ cups chicken broth
Salt and pepper

Heat a medium saucepot. When hot, add the olive oil. Place the onion, celery and carrot in the sauce pot and cook for about 1½-2 minutes until the onions change color and become pale and translucent. Add the thyme, bay leaf and the quinoa and stir to blend mixture completely.

Add the chicken broth and seasonings and stir once or twice, just enough to loosen the quinoa. Bring to a boil, cover with a tight-fitting lid and reduce heat to low. Cook for approximately 18-22 minutes or until all the liquid is absorbed. Remove from the heat and leave covered for at least 5-10 minutes before serving. Makes about 2 cups

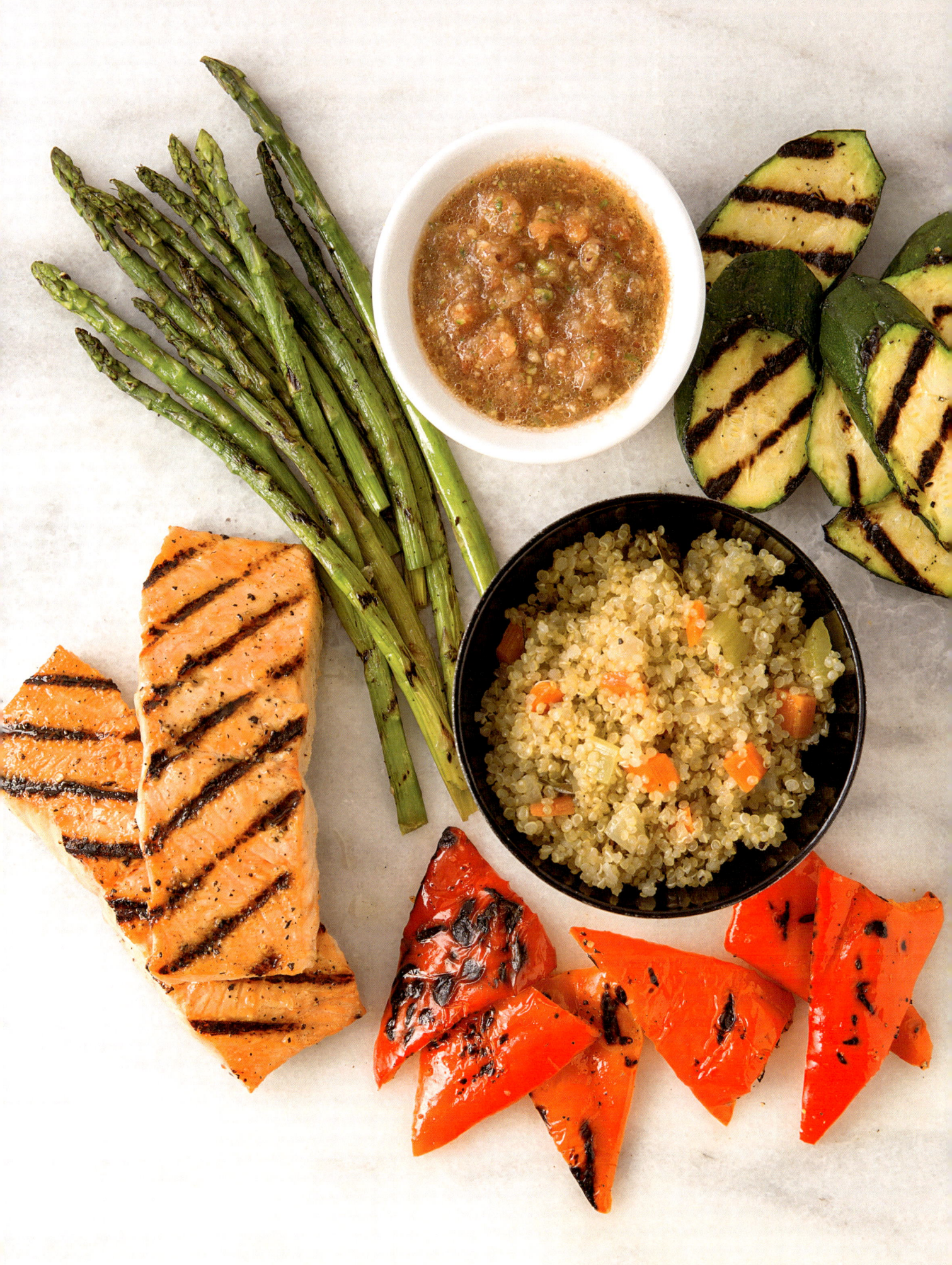

Gazpacho Sauce

1 small zucchini, ends
  trimmed
1 medium red bell
  pepper, stemmed,
  seeded and de-ribbed
½ small red onion,
  peeled
½ small cucumber,
  peeled and seeded
1 clove garlic
2 small tomatoes, peeled,
  seeded, juiced
1 lemon, zested and
  juiced
2 Tbsp olive oil
1 Tbsp stemmed and
  minced fresh oregano
Salt and pepper

Roughly chop the zucchini, bell pepper, onion and cucumber. Place the vegetables, garlic and tomatoes in a food processor and pulse chop until finely minced. Transfer to a mixing bowl and add all the other ingredients. Taste and adjust the seasonings. Set aside. Makes 3 cups

NOTE: Add 1 pint of tomato juice to sauce to make into a refreshing summer soup.

Grilled Vegetables

1 large zucchini
2 red bell peppers
1 lb asparagus, woody
  ends removed
Salt and pepper
2-3 Tbsp olive oil

Wash and trim the ends of the zucchini. Cut the zucchini on a 45° angle in ½-inch slices. Stem, seed and de-rib the bell peppers and cut into 1-inch wide strips.

Heat a grill or cast iron skillet on high heat.

Season the vegetables and brush with olive oil. Place the vegetables across the grates of the grill or in the skillet. Grill the asparagus for approximately 2 minutes per side. Grill the zucchini and the bell pepper for approximately 2-3 minutes per side, then remove all the vegetables. All the vegetables are done when they are slightly bendable. If desired, cut the vegetables smaller after they are grilled.

Grilled Salmon

4 each 4-6 oz salmon
  filets, skinless

Salt and pepper
1-2 Tbsp olive oil

Heat a grill or cast iron skillet on high heat.

Wash the salmon and dry with paper towels. Season both sides of the filets with salt and pepper. Brush with olive oil. Place on the grill and cook for 3-5 minutes on each side, depending on the thickness. Salmon should just be starting to get springy to the touch and not be overcooked, as it will be very dry. Remove and serve.

SERVE THE NEXT DAY COLD

Chili Lime Vinaigrette

¼ cup fresh lime juice
2 Tbsp rice vinegar
1 Tbsp ground cumin
1 Tbsp chili powder
Salt
¾ cup olive oil
Optional, 1 tsp raw
  honey

In a medium mixing bowl, whisk together the lime juice, the rice vinegar, the cumin, the chili powder, and the salt. While whisking, add the oil in a thin stream.

Taste and adjust the seasonings and the balance of the lime juice and olive oil, adding more of either if needed. If desired, raw honey can be added to soften the flavor of the lime juice. Cover and refrigerate until ready to serve. Makes about 1 cup

To Assemble

½ heart of romaine,
  cored and shredded

½ cup Quinoa Pilaf
4-6 Grilled Asparagus
⅓ Grilled Red Bell
  Pepper

2 slices Grilled Zucchini
¼ cup Chili Lime
  Vinaigrette

5-6 oz Grilled Salmon

Pack each ingredient in separate travel containers. When ready to eat, place the romaine in a serving bowl. Top with the quinoa and grilled vegetables. Drizzle with most of the vinaigrette. Top with the salmon and the rest of the vinaigrette. Serve immediately.

SAUTÉED SALMON

This recipe is packed full of "super foods". Wild salmon is more expensive but packs more nutrition than farm-raised salmon. Blueberries boost skin, bone and heart health. Grilling the pineapple caramelizes the fruit. Cooked and shelled edamame can usually be found in the salad bars of most natural food stores.

Make Hot and Fresh
Grilled Pineapple Blueberry Salsa,
Edamame with Almonds, 3 Grain Risotto
Makes 4 Servings

Served The Next Day Cold
Mixed Greens
Makes 1 Serving

3-Grain Risotto

1 Tbsp olive oil
1 small onion, diced
2 cloves garlic, minced
Salt and pepper
½ cup Arborio rice
½ cup quinoa
½ cup quick cooking
   barley
4 cups vegetable stock
⅓ cup grated Parmesan
   cheese

In a large saucepan, heat the oil on medium heat. Add the onion, garlic, salt and pepper. Cook for about 4-5 minutes or until tender, stirring often. Add grains and cook, stirring for 30 seconds. Add the vegetable stock and again bring to a boil. Reduce to a simmer and cover. Cook for 20 minutes or until grains are tender, stirring occasionally. Remove grain mixture from heat. Stir in cheese until melted. Keep covered and warm until ready to serve. Makes about 4 cups

Grilled Pineapple Blueberry Salsa

4 each ½-inch thick slices
   of pineapple, peeled
½ red bell pepper,
   stemmed and seeded
½ red onion, cut in ¼
   inch thick slices
1-2 Tbsp avocado oil
1 tsp chili powder
2 Tbsp minced cilantro
1-2 Tbsp rice wine
   vinegar
1-2 Tbsp lime juice
Salt
¾ cup blueberries, fresh
   or frozen

Heat a grill or cast iron skillet on high heat.

Using the avocado oil, brush both sides of the pineapple, bell pepper and onion slices. Place on the grill and cook the pineapple 60-90 seconds on each side. Continue cooking the onion and bell pepper until soft to the touch, about 3 minutes per side. Remove and let cool.

Remove the core from the pineapple slices, and cut remaining pineapple into ¼-inch dice. Cut the bell pepper into ¼-inch dice. Discard any remaining core from the red onion and cut in ¼-inch dice. Place all in a mixing bowl and add the chili powder, cilantro and half of each of the rice vinegar and lime juice, and mix. Add salt and adjust seasonings, adding more lime juice and rice vinegar as needed. When ready to serve, mix in the blueberries. If not using right away, leave out the berries, cover and refrigerate. Will hold in the refrigerator up to 6 hours. Makes about 2½ cups

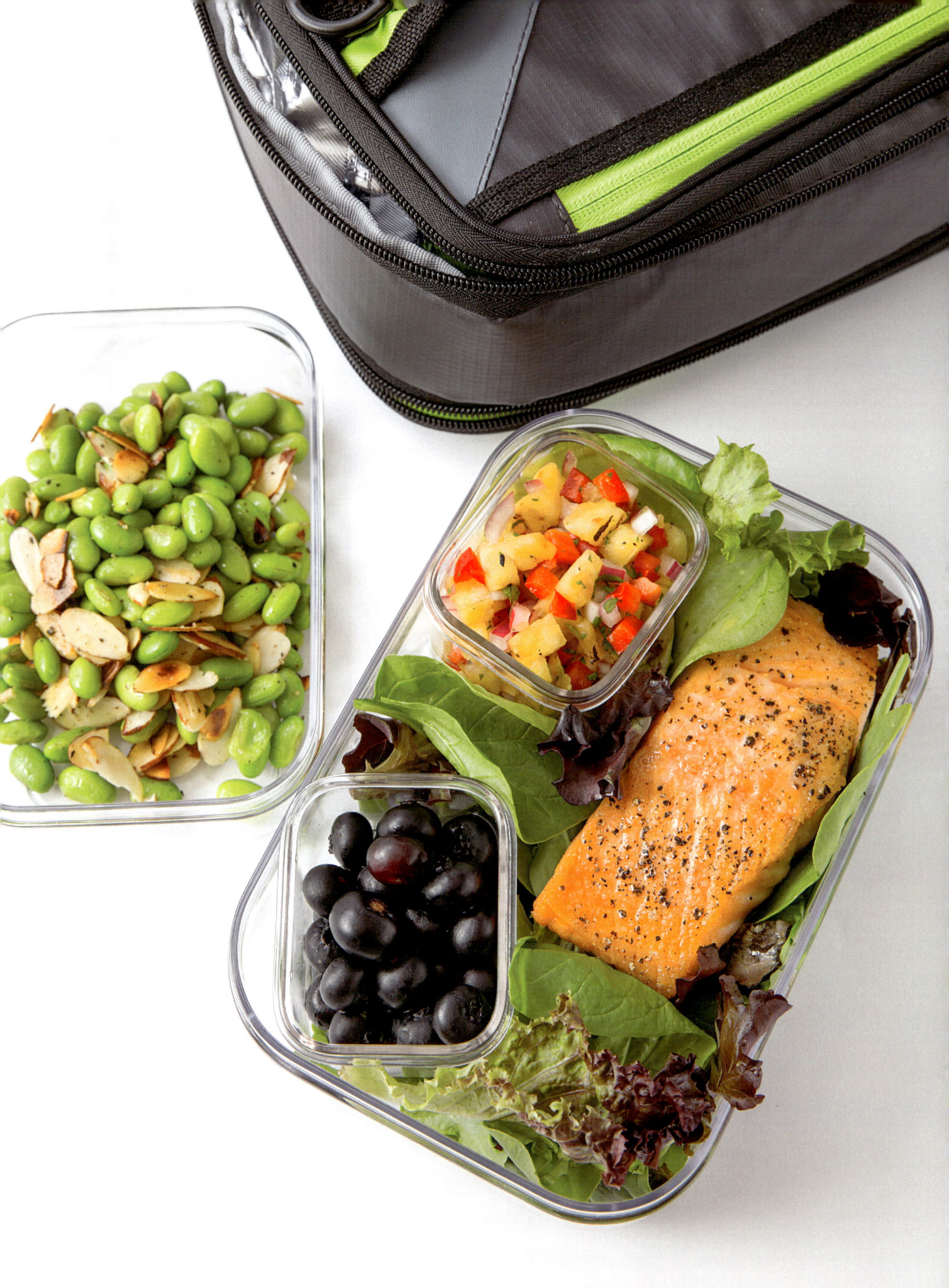

Edamame and Almonds

1 lb edamame, fresh or
  frozen

Salt and pepper
2 Tbsp olive oil
½ cup slivered almonds,
  lightly toasted

Juice of half a lemon

Bring a large pot of salted water to a boil. Add the edamame and bring back to a boil. Cook 5-6 minutes, then drain and place in ice water. When cool, squeeze out the beans from the pods. Set aside. If frozen, thaw and squeeze out the beans.

Heat a medium skillet on medium heat. When hot, add the oil and the beans. Season and cook until hot. Remove from the heat and add the almonds, lemon juice, salt and pepper. Serve immediately.

Sautéed Salmon

4 each 6 oz salmon filets,
  skin on

Salt and pepper
1 Tbsp coconut flour
1-2 Tbsp olive oil

Heat a large skillet on medium high heat.

Rinse and pat dry the salmon. Lightly season the flesh sides of the filets with salt and pepper. Coat the flesh side of the salmon with the coconut flour. Shake off excess.

When the skillet is hot, add the olive oil. Add the salmon and cook 4-5 minutes, then turn over and cook until springy to the touch. Total cooking time should be 10-12 minutes per inch of thickness.

SERVE THE NEXT DAY COLD

2 oz mixed greens
1 Sautéed Salmon Filet
⅓ cup Edamame and
  Almonds
⅓ Grilled Pineapple
  Blueberry Salsa
1 heaping Tbsp
  blueberries, fresh or
  frozen

Pack each ingredient in separate travel containers. Just prior to eating, place the salmon on the greens, top with edamame and salsa and garnish with blueberries.

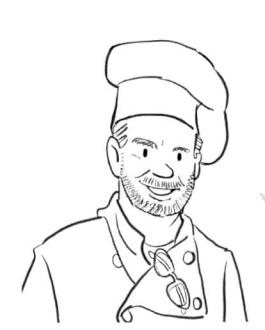

Measurements are truly personal — I have always used the rule that a pinch of salt is three fingers worth, but you might develop your own, depending upon your taste.

ARTICHOKE AND CHÈVRE FRITTATA

When it comes to ingredients in a frittata, one of my favorite sayings is, "You are only limited by your imagination." This easy egg dish is great for breakfast, brunch or a late night supper, and the potatoes complete the meal.

Make Hot and Fresh
Baby Red Potato Hash with
Fresh Herbs and Garlic
Makes 4 Servings

Serve The Next Day Hot
Makes 1 Serving

Baby Red Potato Hash with Fresh Herbs and Garlic

2 lbs small red potatoes, ¼-inch dice

Salt and pepper

3 Tbsp olive oil, or as needed

2 Tbsp chopped shallots

2 tsp minced garlic

1 Tbsp stemmed and minced rosemary

1 Tbsp stemmed and minced thyme

Place the potatoes in a large pot and cover with cold water, then add salt. Bring to a boil and cook for about 3 minutes. Remove and drain, then let cool and air dry.

Heat the oil in a large skillet, add potatoes, then season with salt and pepper. Let brown before stirring, then stir occasionally, until potatoes are tender to the bite. Finish with shallots, garlic and rosemary and thyme. Keep warm until ready to serve.

Artichoke Chèvre Frittata

3 Tbsp butter

½ zucchini, diced

½ red bell pepper, diced

½ cup diced green beans

2 shallots, diced

1 clove garlic minced

Salt and pepper

½ can artichoke hearts, drained and chopped

8 eggs, beaten

3 oz chèvre (goat) cheese, crumbled

Preheat oven to 425°F.

Heat a 12-inch nonstick pan on medium heat. When hot, add the butter and the zucchini, bell pepper and green beans. Cook for about 4 minutes, or until almost tender, then add the shallots, garlic, salt and pepper. Cook another 1-2 minutes to soften the shallots.

Add the artichokes and eggs, and then top with the cheese. Place in the oven until eggs are set and lightly puffed, about 8-12 minutes. Remove and cut into 4 wedges and serve.

SERVE THE NEXT DAY HOT

1 wedge Artichoke
Chèvre Frittata

1-1½ cups Baby Red
Potato Hash

Place the frittata and the potatoes in separate microwave-proof travel containers. When ready to eat, sprinkle 1 Tbsp water on top of the frittata, loosely place the lids on and reheat for 3-4 minutes.

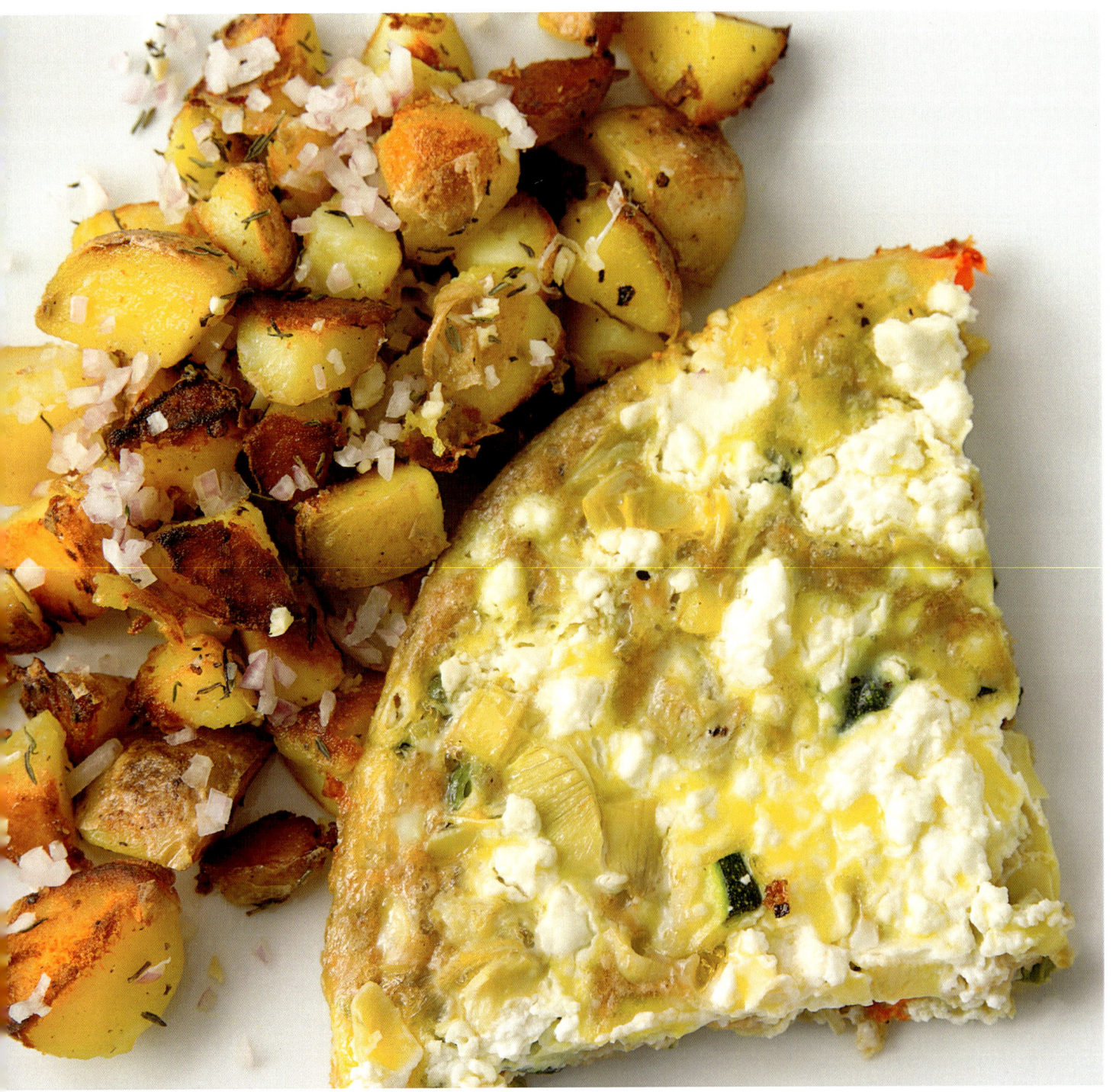

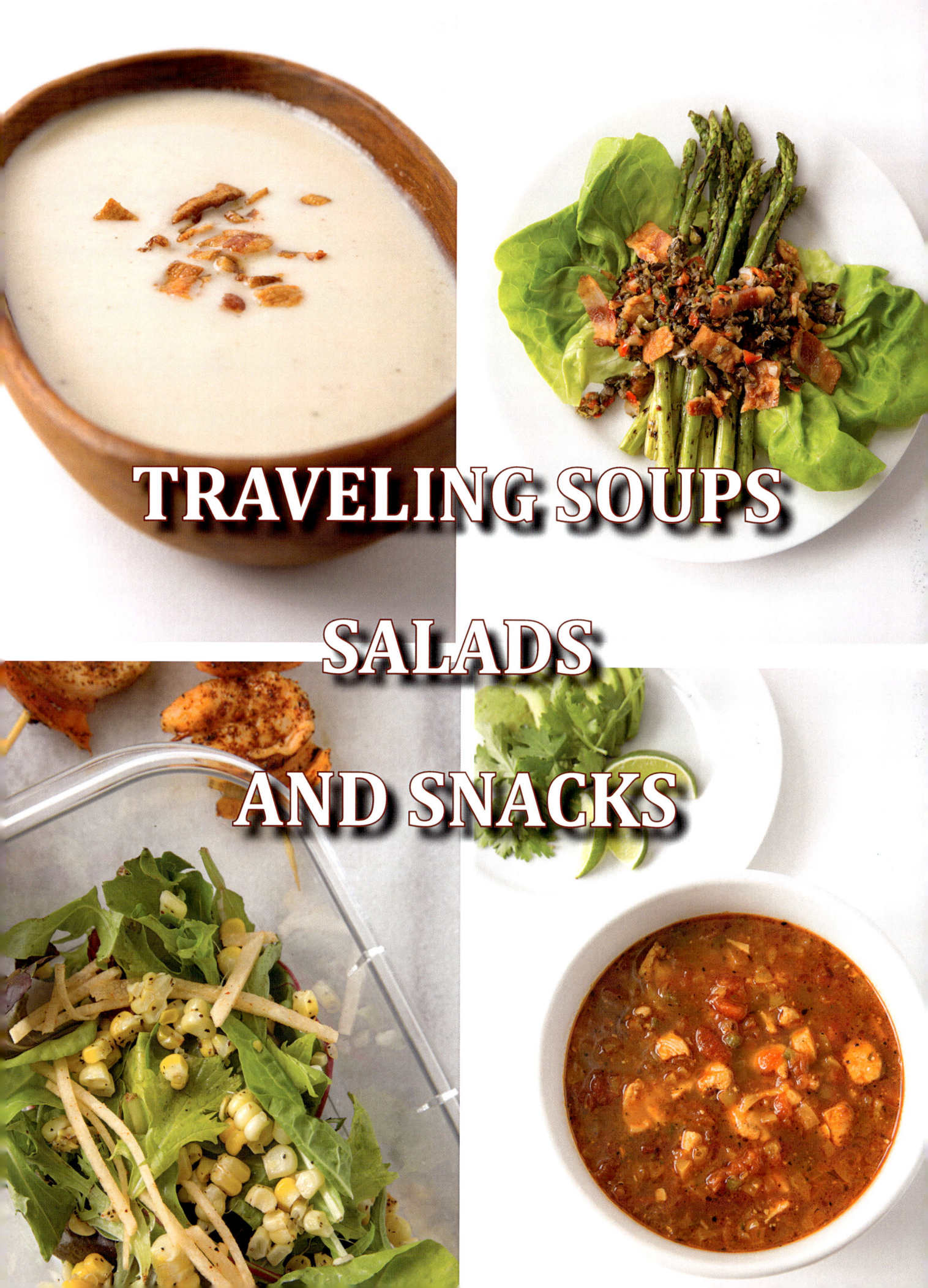

TRAVELING SOUPS

SALADS

AND SNACKS

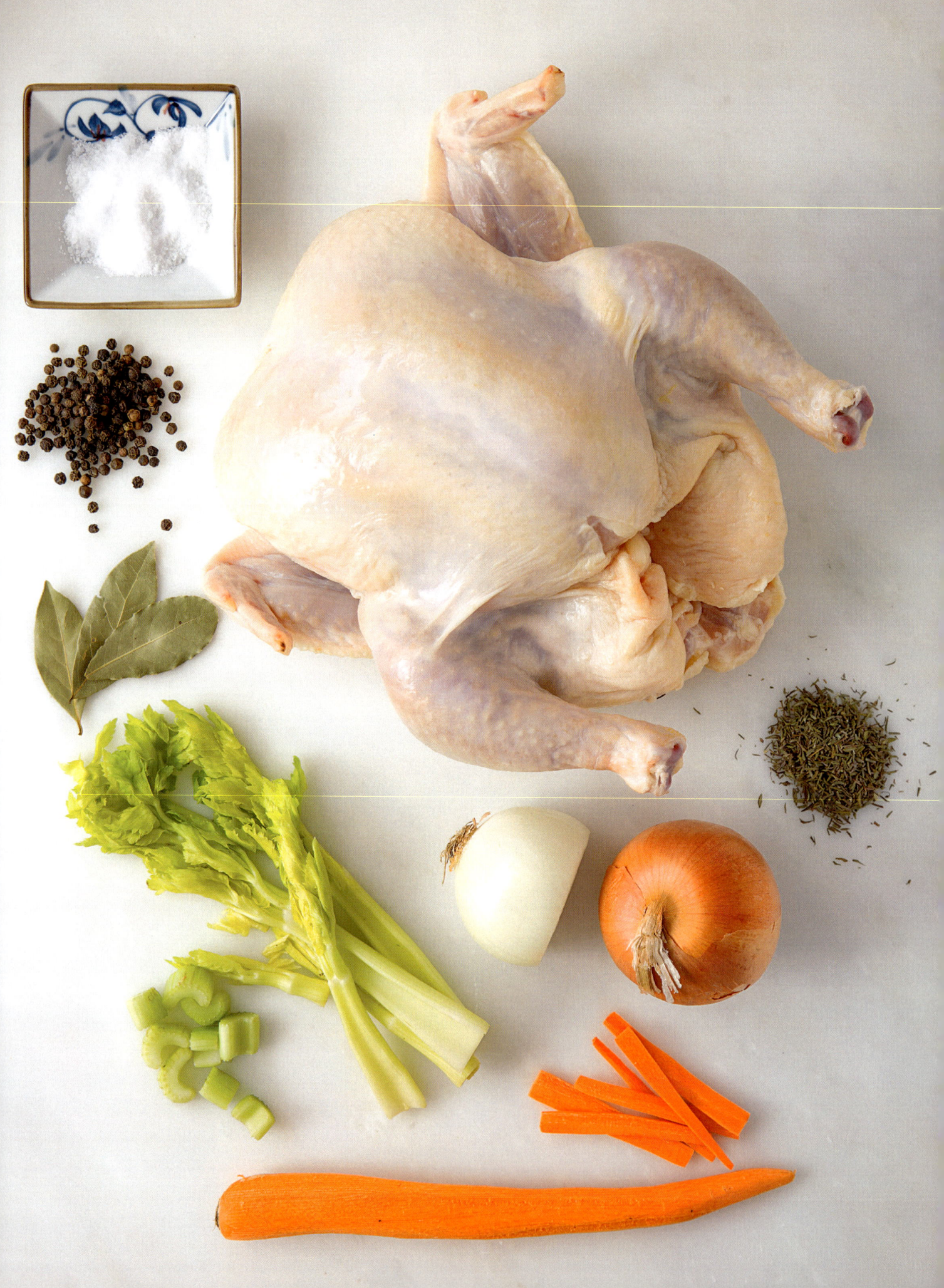

BASIC CHICKEN STOCK

The hardest part of making stock is learning what not to do. First, never stir. Second, never boil. All minor impurities will float to the surface and can be removed by skimming with a ladle. Stirring and boiling pushes these minor impurities back into the stock. This "scum" is in no way bad for you or the stock but removing it will yield a cleaner and clearer finished product. After the stock is strained, it can be boiled and stirred.

Makes about 1 gallon

5 lbs chicken bones
1 lb chicken feet, if available
2 carrots, trimmed and chopped
1 large onion, peeled and chopped
2 celery stalks, trimmed and chopped
2 bay leaves
10-12 whole black peppercorns
2 Tbsp dried thyme
Cold water to cover bones by 1-2 inches, approximately 6 quarts

Rinse and remove the fat and blood from the bones and feet.

Add all the ingredients to a large stockpot. The water should cover the bones by 1-2 inches. Bring to boiling temperature, uncovered, without actually allowing the stock to boil. Reduce to a simmer and, using a ladle, skim off any foam that rises to the surface.

Simmer very slowly for 2½-3 hours, skimming the foam as needed.

Using a fine mesh sieve or colander, strain the stock into a large pot. Let cool, stirring occasionally, for at least 30 minutes and up to an hour. Loosely cover to allow the stock to continue to cool and refrigerate with a small wire rack underneath. This allows the cool air to circulate around the pot.

NOTE: Any unskimmed fat will congeal at the top of the stock during refrigeration. Remove this fat prior to usage.

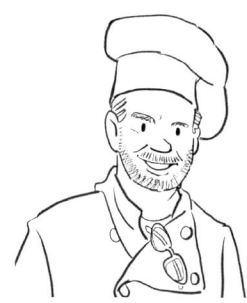

This chicken stock can also be made with the leftover carcasses from your roasted chicken(s). Stocks freeze well without losing their quality, too.

ITALIAN WEDDING SOUP
Sausage Meatballs

This soup follows the traditional procedure of cooking soup on the stove – bringing the ingredients to a boil – which means it reaches its desired temperature quickly and efficiently - and then reducing to a simmer while covering – a slower and more steady method, which offers control and ensures even cooking.

Makes 6-8 Servings

Sausage Meatballs

½ lb chicken sausage, casings removed

½ lb mild bulk Italian pork sausage

⅔ cup gluten-free breadcrumbs

2 cloves garlic, minced

3 Tbsp chopped fresh parsley

1 extra-large egg, lightly beaten

Salt and pepper

Preheat the oven to 350°F.

Place the ground chicken, pork sausage, breadcrumbs, garlic, parsley, egg, salt and pepper in a large mixing bowl and combine well. With a teaspoon, drop 1 to 1¼-inch meatballs onto a sheet pan lined with parchment paper. Lightly oil your hands and then gently roll each meatball into a round ball. Place in the oven and bake for about 15 minutes, or until springy to the touch. Remove and set aside.

Italian Wedding Soup

2 Tbsp olive oil

1 cup diced yellow onion

1 cup diced carrots

¾ cup diced celery

Optional, ½ cup dry white wine

10 cups chicken stock, preferably homemade, see recipe page 107

3 cups cooked basmati rice

3 Tbsp minced fresh oregano

12 oz baby spinach or chopped escarole, washed

Sausage Meatballs, cooked

Heat a large soup pot on high heat. When hot, add the olive oil. Add the onion, carrots, and celery and sauté for 2-3 minutes until softened, stirring occasionally. Add the wine, if using, and bring to a full boil, then add the chicken stock and return to a boil. Reduce to a simmer and cook for about 10-15 minutes, or until the vegetables are tender.

Add the rice, oregano, spinach or escarole and cooked meatballs to the broth and bring to a simmer. Taste and adjust the seasonings. Ladle the soup into serving bowls.

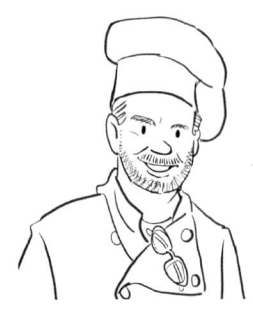

Seasonings are always to taste – never to measurement. Always remember to taste your food as you go, so you can add seasonings to your liking. Most people under-season their food, so don't be shy with the salt and pepper.

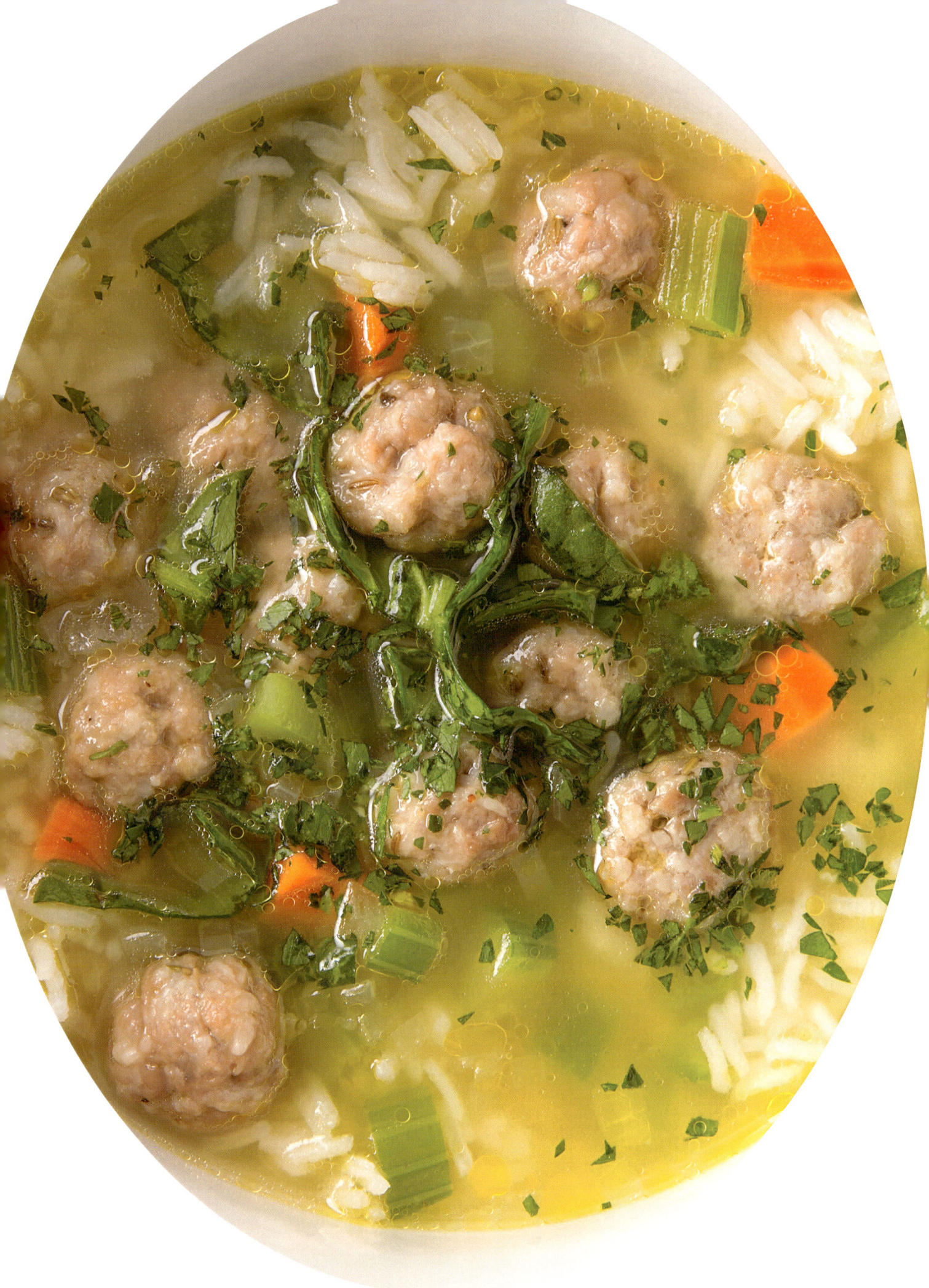

TORTILLA SOUP
Fresh Lime and Avocado
Makes 6 Servings

2 Tbsp olive oil

1 yellow onion, diced

3 cloves garlic, minced

2 jalapeños, stemmed, seeded and minced

6-7 cups chicken stock preferably homemade, see recipe page 107

1 each 14.5-oz can fire-roasted diced tomatoes

1 each 14.5-oz can black beans, rinsed and drained

Salt and pepper

3 chicken breasts, boneless and skinless

2 limes, juiced, plus wedges for garnish

1 cup roughly chopped fresh cilantro leaves

1 small bag organic corn tortilla chips, hand crumbled

1 avocado, pitted, sliced

Heat a large soup pot on medium-high heat and when hot, add the oil. Add the onions and cook for about 2-3 minutes, or until the onions become translucent. Add the garlic and jalapeños and cook for another minute. Add the chicken stock, tomatoes, beans, salt and pepper and bring to a boil.

Add the chicken breasts, bring to a simmer and cook for about 20-25 minutes, or until the chicken breasts are firm to the touch. Remove the chicken and let cool. When cool enough to handle, chop or hand tear into small, bite-sized pieces. Return to the soup, and bring to a simmer. Taste and adjust the seasonings. Keep warm until ready to serve.

When ready to serve, add lime juice and fresh cilantro to the pot. Taste and adjust the seasonings. In a serving bowl add a mound of the chicken. Ladle soup over the chicken and serve with lime wedge, tortilla strips, and avocado slices.

Although this soup is delicious on its own, I'd recommend serving bowls full of grated cheese, fresh or pickled jalapeños, sour cream, slices of avocado and lime quarters. All essential accompaniments, in my opinion!

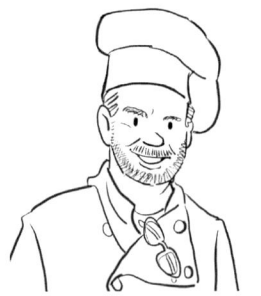

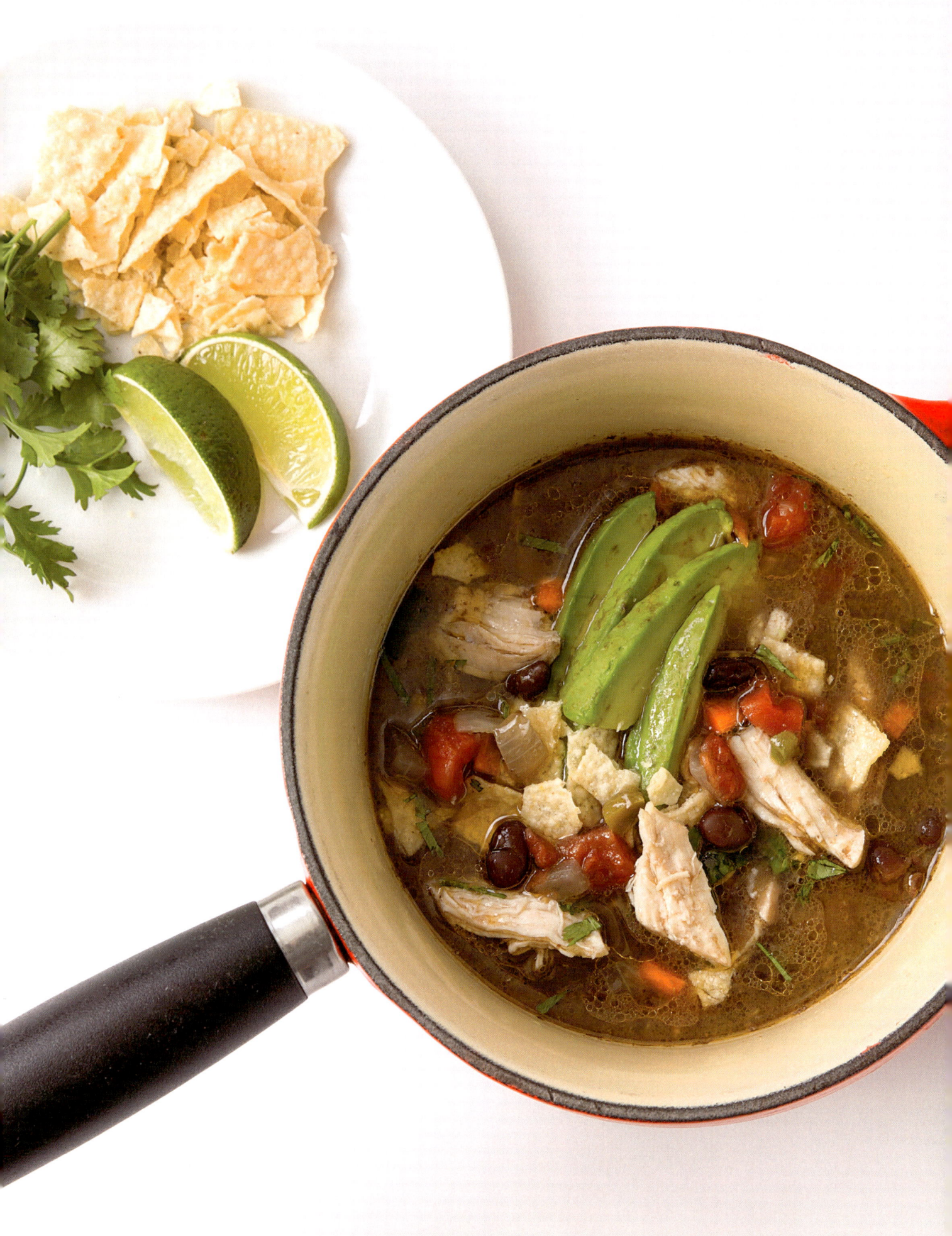

CAULIFLOWER SOUP
Apple, Dijon and Hazelnut Garnish
Makes 6-8 Servings

Cauliflower Soup

2 leeks
3 strips bacon, diced
2 Tbsp olive oil
1 celery rib, with extra leaves, coarsely chopped
Salt and pepper
2 Tbsp finely minced garlic
Pinch nutmeg
6 cups chicken stock, preferably homemade, see recipe page 107 or vegetable stock
Juice of half a lemon
1 head cauliflower, cored and broken into florets
1 cup extra-soft tofu, diced

Trim the green from the top of the leeks and cut in half lengthwise. Wash to remove dirt. Pat dry and thinly slice crosswise.

Heat a large soup pot on medium heat, and when hot, add the bacon and cook until it begins to brown. Pour off excess bacon fat. Add the oil, leeks, celery with leaves and salt and pepper. Cook for about 4 minutes, or until softened, then add the garlic and nutmeg and cook for another 30 seconds. Add the stock, lemon juice, and cauliflower florets. Raise the heat to high and bring to a boil, then reduce to a simmer and cook for about 15 minutes, or until the cauliflower is very tender. Add the tofu.

Purée in a blender in batches until very smooth. Transfer to a soup pot. Taste and adjust the seasonings. Add extra broth for desired consistency. Keep warm until ready to serve.

Apple Dijon and Hazelnut Garnish

1 Tbsp grapeseed oil
1 firm apple, peeled, cored and diced
1 Tbsp Dijon mustard
¼ cup coarsely chopped hazelnuts

Heat a skillet on medium heat. When hot, add the oil and apples. Cook for about 4 minutes until soft. Add the Dijon and toss to coat the apples. Remove and let cool, then stir in the hazelnuts. Set aside.

To Serve

Ladle hot soup into soup bowls, place a heaping tablespoon of the garnish in the center and serve.

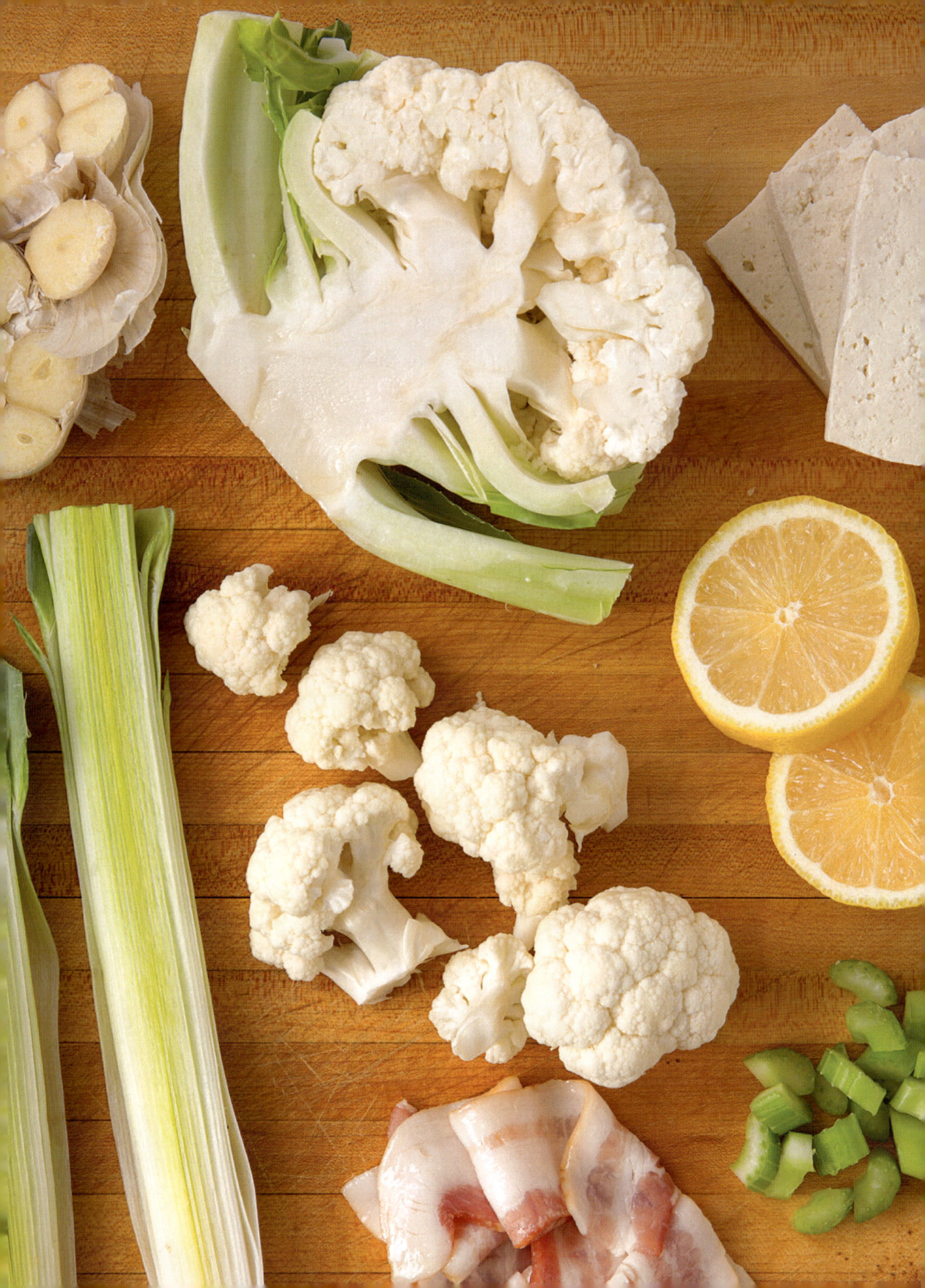

JODIE'S CHICKEN FAJITA SOUP
Makes 6-8 Servings

This recipe comes from my terrific assistant Jodie Leschuk who made it as part of a fun contest we had with my staff at The Seasoned Chef and The Gourmet Spoon. The competition was lively and this soup was the winner. It is as delicious as it is healthy and satisfying.

8 medium tomatoes
3 Tbsp chili powder
1 Tbsp paprika
1 Tbsp cumin
2 red bell peppers, diced
2 green bell peppers, diced
2 jalapeños, diced
2 poblano peppers, diced
2 small onions, diced
Salt and pepper
2 lbs boneless skinless chicken thighs, cut into ½-inch dice
Avocado oil
3 cloves garlic, minced
5-7 cups chicken stock, preferably homemade, see recipe page 107
2 tsp Tabasco, or to taste
Optional, diced avocado, lime wedges, stemmed and minced cilantro, for garnish

Preheat oven to 400°F.

Wash the tomatoes and cut in half. Squeeze out the seeds with your hand and place cut side down on a parchment lined sheet pan. Place in the oven and roast for 15-20 minutes or until very soft. Remove, let cool, dice and set aside.

Mix the chili powder, paprika and cumin together and divide in half. Place the peppers and onions together in a medium mixing bowl and toss with half of the spice mixture. Add salt and pepper. In a separate bowl, toss the chicken with the other half of spice mixture. Add salt and pepper.

Heat a large soup pot on medium heat. When hot, add enough oil to coat the bottom of the pan. In batches, sauté first the chicken thighs and then the peppers and onions, making sure to pick up browned pieces of chicken off the bottom of the pan. Once the vegetables are cooked, return the chicken to the pan. Add the garlic, roasted tomatoes, chicken stock and Tabasco. Bring the soup to a boil and reduce to a simmer for about 20-25 minutes, skimming the fat occasionally. Taste and adjust seasonings.

When ready to serve, if desired, prepare bowls of diced avocados, lime wedges and cilantro.

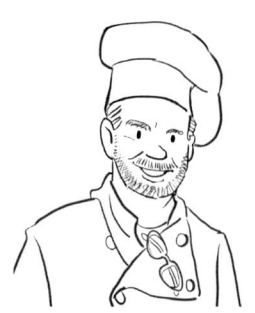

Although fresh cilantro is an authentic garnish here, 1 in 7 people think it tastes like soap (!) so it is easily added or omitted.

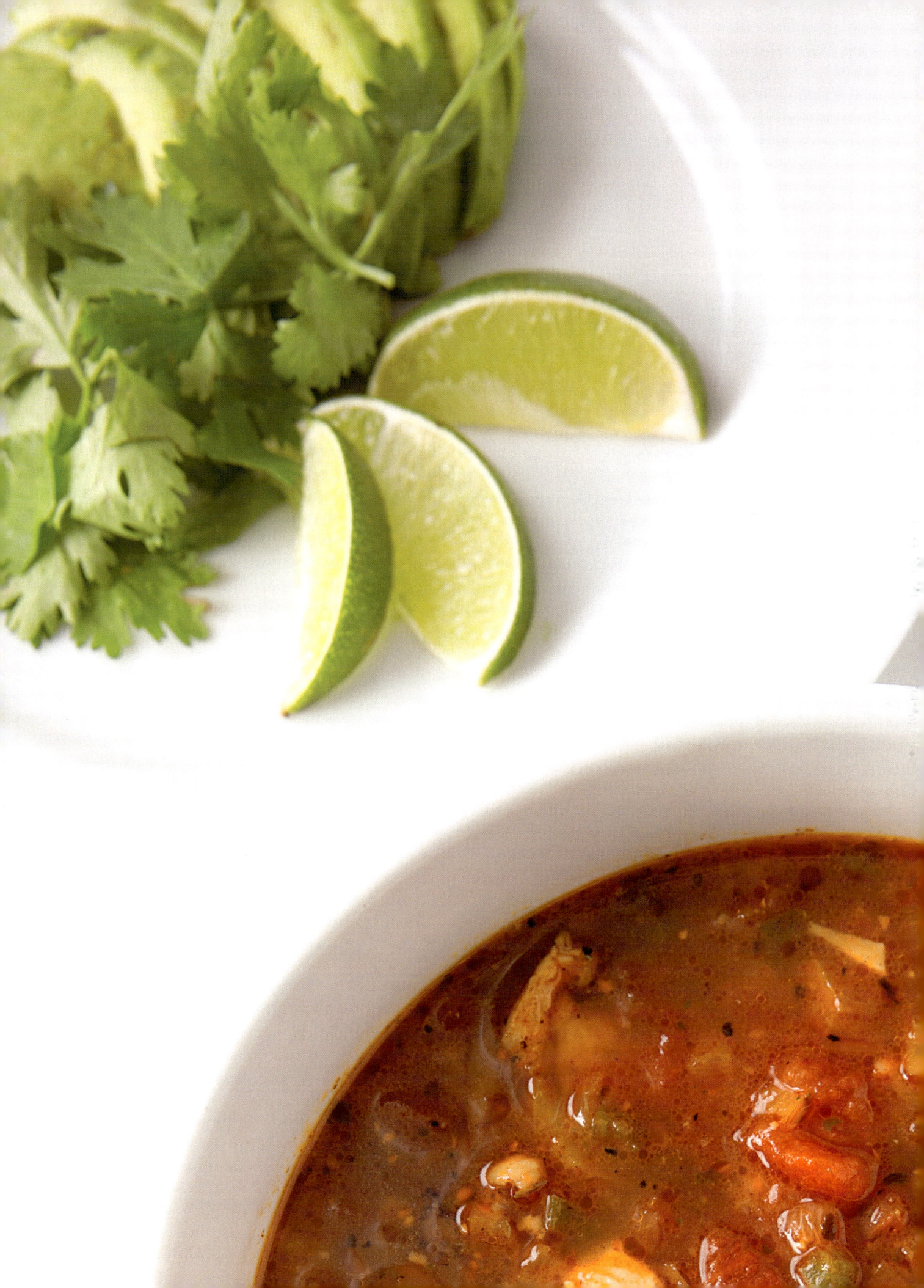

HOT SMOKED SALMON SALAD
Lemon Caper Vinaigrette, Arugula and Fennel
Makes 4 Servings

Hot Smoked Salmon

4 each 5-oz salmon filets, skin on

Salt and pepper

Optional, 1 Tbsp green or black tea leaves

Applewood, cherry or wine-soaked oak wood chips

Prepare a smoker according to manufacturer's instructions. Place the salmon skin side down on the smoker rack. Season with salt and pepper. If desired, sprinkle tea leaves directly onto the wood chips. This will impart a slightly different flavor and aroma to the finished product. Place the rack in the smoker, cover with the lid and smoke for approximately 15-20 minutes after the first signs of smoke appear. Salmon is done when it is slightly firm to the touch.

Lemon Caper Vinaigrette

2 Tbsp fresh lemon juice
2 Tbsp rice wine vinegar
2 Tbsp minced chives
Salt and pepper
¾ cup olive oil
2 Tbsp drained capers

Mix the lemon juice, rice vinegar, chives, salt and pepper together with a wire whip. Whisk in the olive oil. Add the capers, adjust seasonings and set aside. May be made one day ahead. Makes about 1 cup

To Assemble

5 oz arugula
2 cups thinly sliced fennel bulb
½ cup thinly sliced red onion
¼ cup oil-packed sun-dried tomatoes, julienned
¾ cup Lemon Caper Vinaigrette
4 Hot Smoked Salmon filets

Arrange the salad ingredients on a platter and drizzle with the dressing. Remove the skin from the salmon and place on the salad.

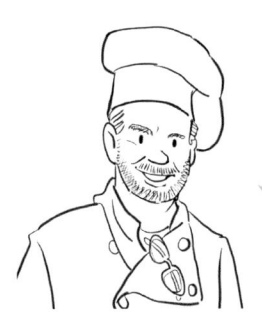

Proper knife skills are imperative when cooking fresh food – I encourage everyone to enroll in a cooking class to learn the correct way to chop, mince and julienne. It is the best cooking investment you can make!

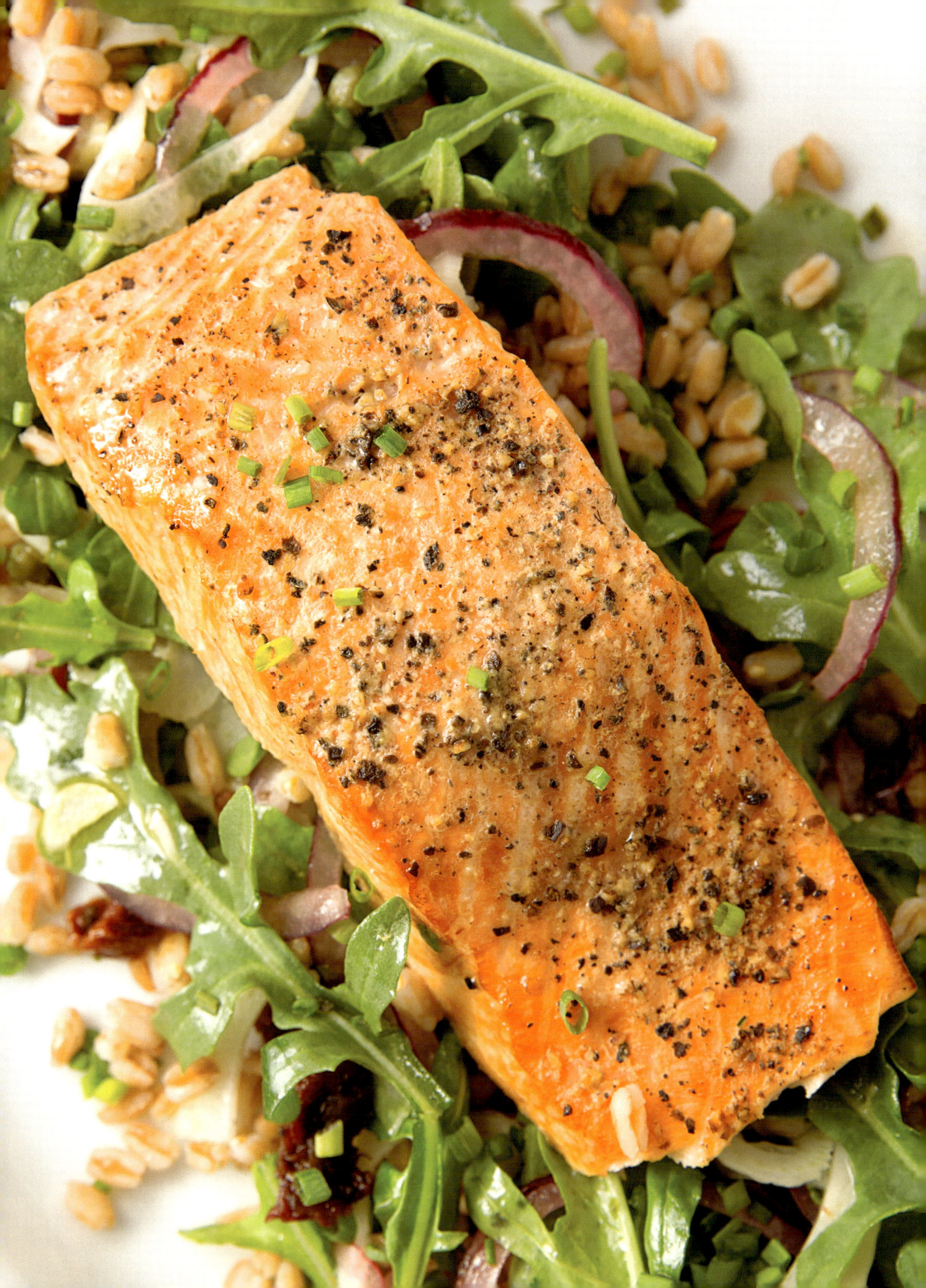

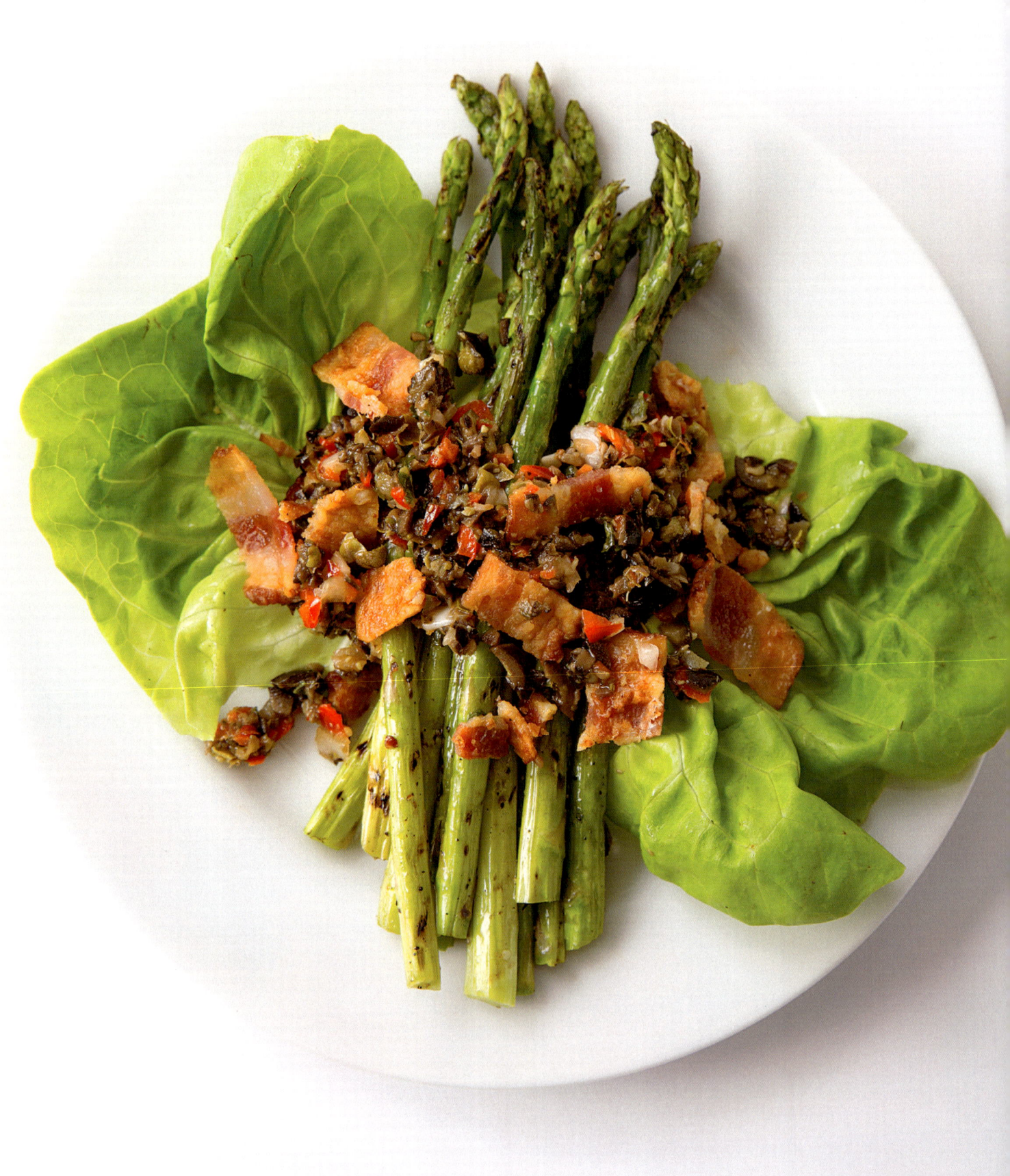

GRILLED ASPARAGUS WITH SMOKED BACON
AND BLACK OLIVE CAPER TAPENADE
Makes 4 Servings

Grilled Asparagus

1 lb medium asparagus
 spears, woody ends
 removed

Salt and pepper
2 Tbsp olive oil

Heat a grill or cast iron skillet to high heat.

Season and oil the asparagus spears. Lay the spears across the grates of the grill rack. Grill the asparagus for approximately 1½-2 minutes on each side, or until bendable to the touch. Remove and let cool.

Black Olive Caper Tapenade

½ cup cured black olives,
 pits removed, chopped

2 Tbsp capers, chopped
1 shallot, minced
½ red bell pepper,
 minced

1 clove garlic, minced
1 Tbsp lemon juice
1 Tbsp white vinegar
1 Tbsp chopped fresh
 basil

4-6 Tbsp olive oil
Salt and pepper
Optional, 2-3 anchovy
 filets, finely chopped

Blend all ingredients together, taste and adjust the seasonings. Alternately, you may also place all ingredients in a food processor, prior to mincing and chopping, and pulse chop until blended. Makes about 1½ cups

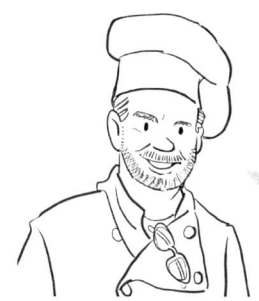

Although the base of this rich and full-flavored spread is olives, don't omit the capers here. The word 'tapenade' actually comes from the Provençal word for capers, 'tapanas', and their unique pickled tang is essential here.

To Assemble

1 head butter lettuce,
 washed and leaves
 separated

6 oz applewood smoked
 bacon, cooked and
 chopped

Lay the lettuce leaves on a platter. Top with the asparagus, tapenade and bacon.

For the next day, use the lettuce leaves as a wrap for the other components.

MEDITERRANEAN CHOPPED SALAD
Red Wine Vinaigrette
Makes 8-10 Servings

Red Wine Vinaigrette

⅓ cup red wine
vinaigrette

2 Tbsp Dijon mustard

2 cloves garlic, minced

Salt and pepper

1 cup olive oil

Optional, ⅓ cup freshly
grated Parmesan
cheese

In a medium mixing bowl, whisk together the vinegar, mustard, garlic, salt and pepper.

Gradually whisk in the oil in a slow, steady stream until well blended. (You can also make this in the blender.) Mix in the Parmesan cheese. Taste and adjust seasonings, if necessary. Refrigerate in a covered container. Makes about 1½ cups

Mediterranean Chopped Salad

4 large tomatoes,
chopped

2 medium cucumbers,
peeled, seeded and
chopped

1 medium red onion,
finely chopped

1 red bell pepper,
coarsely chopped

1 green bell pepper,
coarsely chopped

1 carrot, peeled and
diced

1 zucchini, diced

½ cup Italian parsley,
coarsely chopped

½ cup olives, any kind,
pitted and sliced

Optional, ½ cup chopped
ham, salami, prosciutto,
etc.

In a large bowl, combine all the ingredients. Add about ¾ cup dressing and toss well. Add more dressing as needed. Taste and adjust the seasonings. Transfer to a platter and serve immediately.

NOTE: You can use a wide variety of vegetables and cooked meats in this salad. The recipe here is a mere template.

All salads travel well, and should be dressed just before eating. If the salad has delicate leafy greens, always toss those with the dressing before serving.

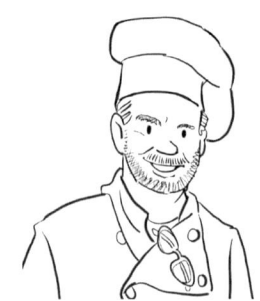

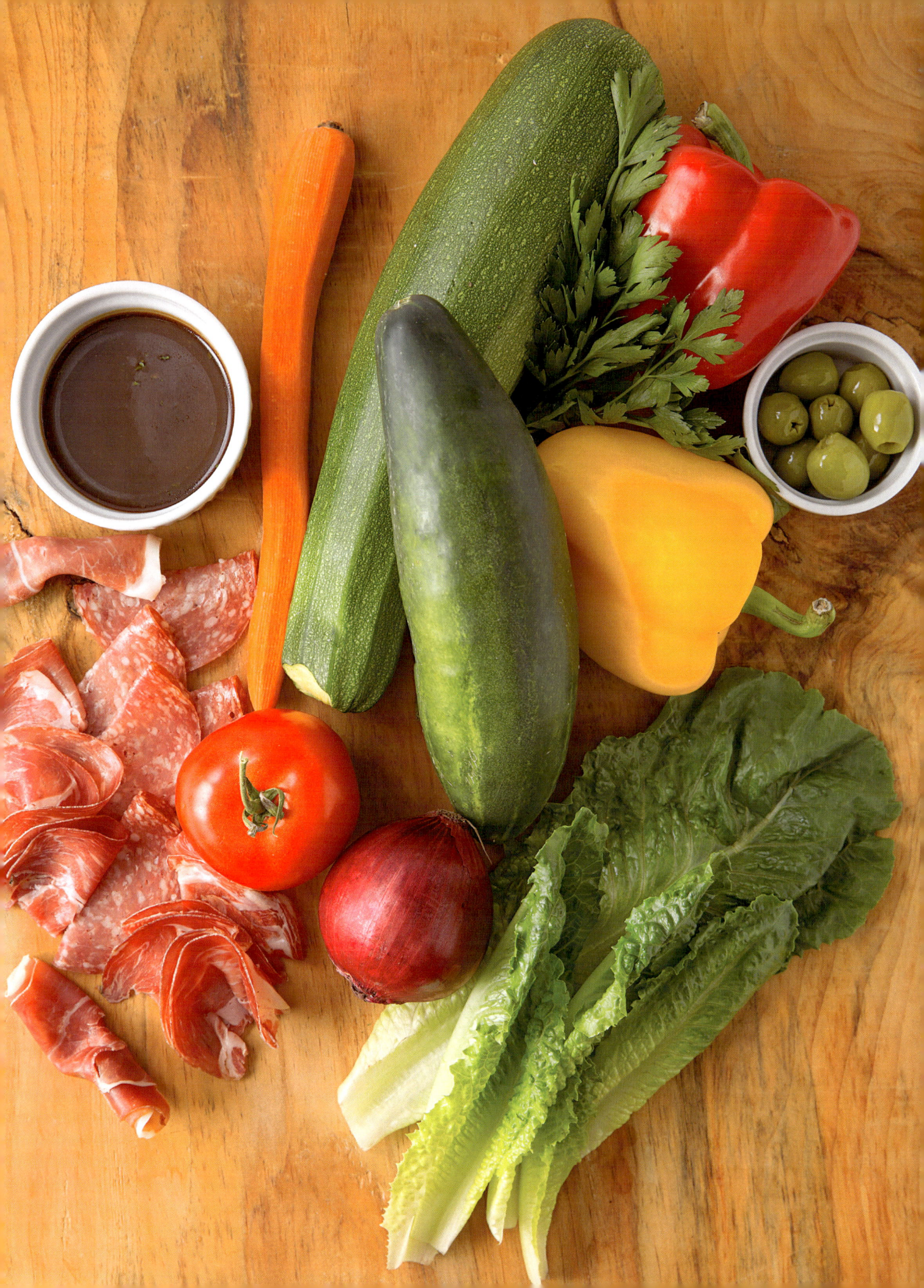

TRAVELING CAESAR SALAD

Caesar Dressing

2 cloves garlic, peeled
1 anchovy fillet
1 Tbsp Dijon mustard
2-3 tsp Worcestershire
    sauce
1-2 Tbsp lemon juice
Tabasco, to taste
Freshly ground black
    pepper
⅓ cup olive oil

In a food processer, place the garlic, anchovy, Dijon mustard, Worcestershire sauce, lemon juice, Tabasco and pepper. Purée, then with the motor running, slowly pour in the olive oil. Taste and adjust the seasonings. Makes about ½ cup

Salad

2 hearts of romaine,
    cored and sliced thin or
    any Spring lettuce mix
4 green onions, cleaned
    and sliced on a 45°
    angle
1 cup cherry tomatoes,
    any kind
½ cucumber, peeled and
    thinly sliced
1 can dark red kidney
    beans, drained and
    rinsed
1 avocado, diced
Optional, ⅓ cup grated
    Parmesan cheese
Optional, ¾ cup roasted
    and salted corn kernels

When ready to eat, toss together all ingredients except the corn, top with dressing and garnish with corn kernels. Reserve any remaining undressed vegetables and dressing for the next day.

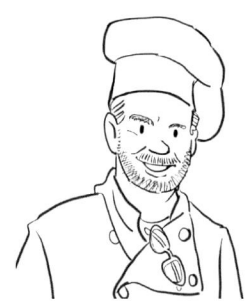

Avocados are a terrific addition to almost any salad; however, if they are served in a traveling dish, they need to travel whole and then be split, seeded and cut just before serving.

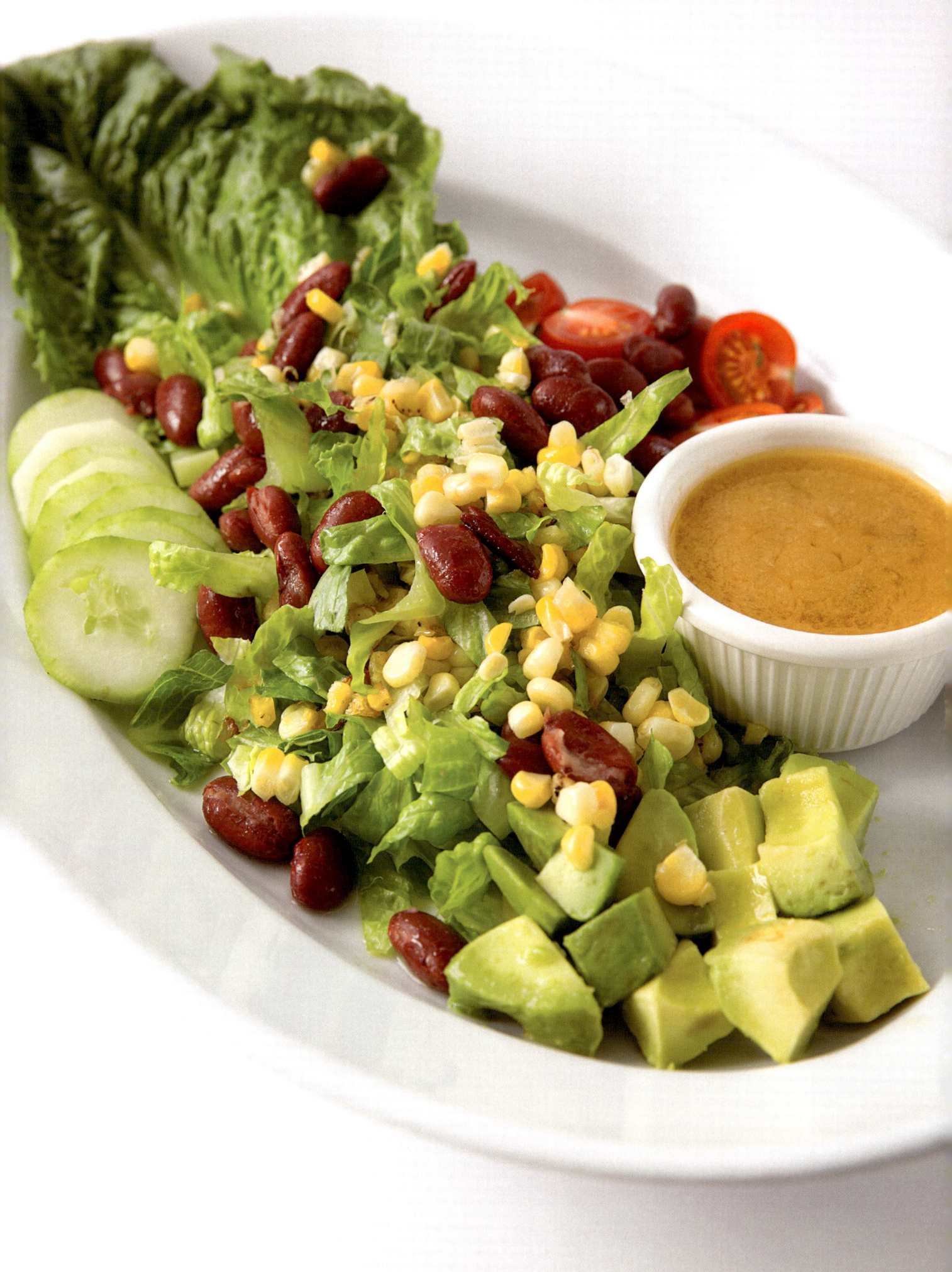

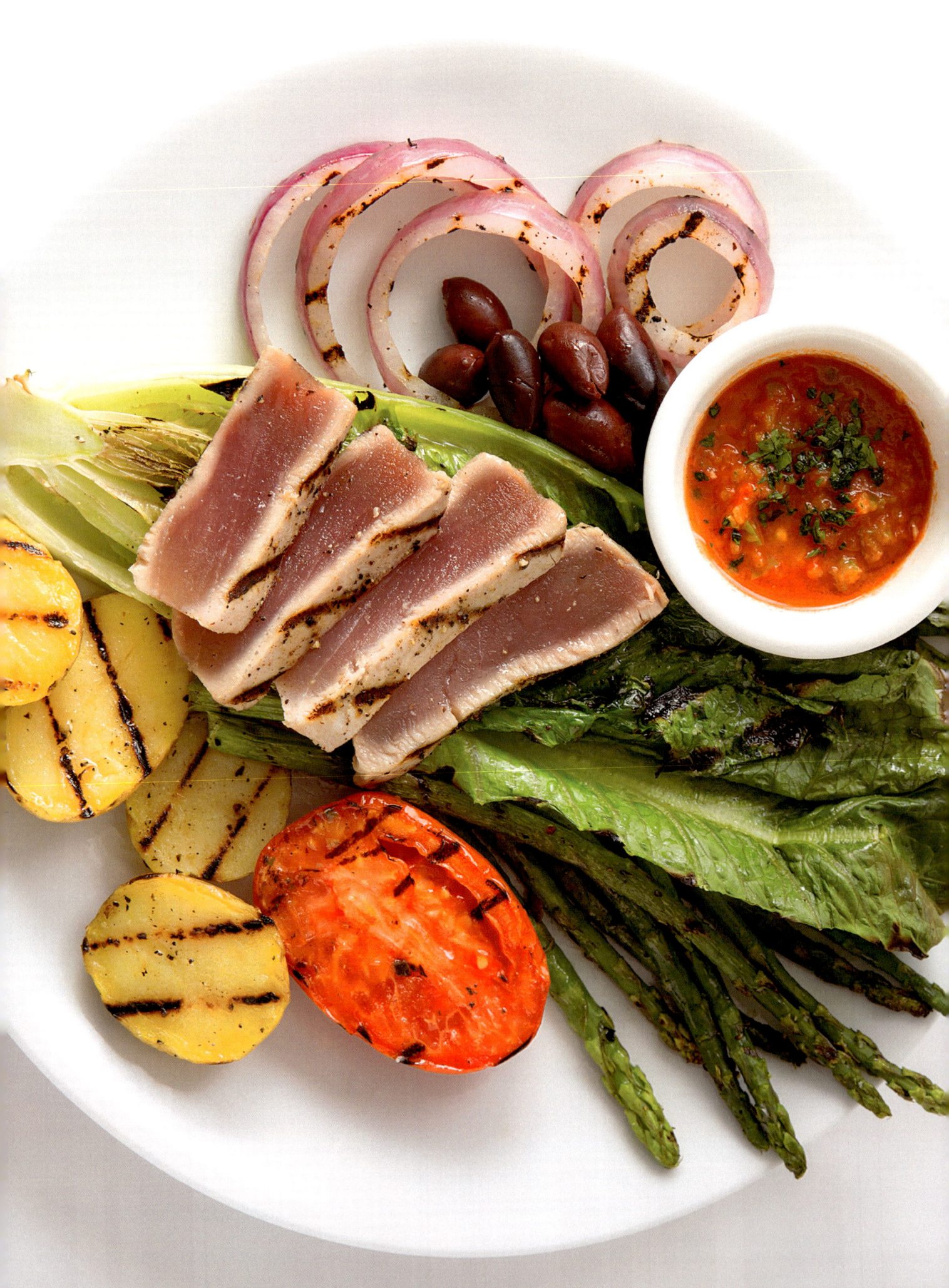

GRILLED TUNA NIÇOISE SALAD
Roasted Tomato Vinaigrette

Quite simply one of my favorite salads, and one which I frequently feature in classes at my cooking school. The recipe involves making an emulsified vinaigrette, proper cooking of a variety of fresh vegetables, and the correct way to cook a delicate protein. A fun way to serve this on Day 1 is to lay all the components out, and have your family or friends compose their own customized plate.

Makes 4 Servings

Roasted Tomato Vinaigrette

2 medium tomatoes, cut in half

Salt and pepper
1 Tbsp olive oil
1 shallot, peeled and chopped

2 cloves garlic
1 Tbsp tomato paste
3 Tbsp red wine vinegar
1 Tbsp lemon juice
½ cup olive oil
2 Tbsp stemmed and minced basil

Preheat oven to 400°F.

Season the cut side of the tomatoes with salt and pepper, then place them cut side down on a sheet pan. Lightly brush the skins with olive oil. Put the tomatoes in the oven and cook for about 20 minutes, until very soft. Remove, let cool, then remove the skins.

Place the tomatoes, shallots, garlic, salt and pepper, tomato paste, vinegar, and lemon juice into a food processor and puree until smooth. With the motor still running, slowly add the olive oil. Transfer to a serving bowl and add the basil. Taste and adjust the seasonings. Makes about 1½ cups

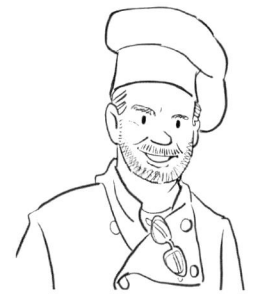

Grilling your Romaine takes this salad to a whole new level — smoky and charred, it adds both flavor and texture to the dish.

Grilled Tuna Niçoise Salad

6 small new potatoes
¼ cup olive oil or more
  as needed
Salt and pepper
1 bunch asparagus,
  woody ends removed

2 Roma tomatoes
1 medium red onion
2 hearts of romaine
2 each 8 oz tuna steaks
½ cup Niçoise olives

Preheat grill or cast iron skillet.

Put the potatoes in a pot of cold water, bring to a boil and cook for about 15 minutes, or until al dente. Cool and split in half. Brush with olive oil, then season with salt and pepper. Grill for about 3-4 minutes on cut side only. Set aside.

Lay out the asparagus, brush with olive oil, then season with salt and pepper. Grill for about 2-3 minutes, then turn over and continue to cook for 2-3 more minutes until tender to the bite, depending on the thickness of the asparagus. Set aside.

Core and split the Roma tomatoes in half. Brush with olive oil, then season with salt and pepper. Grill for 30-40 seconds on cut side only. Set aside.

Peel the red onion, core and cut into ½-inch thick slices. Brush with olive oil, then season with salt and pepper. Grill slices for 3-4 minutes on each side. Set aside.

Wash and trim the hearts of romaine, leaving the core intact and split in half lengthwise. Lightly oil the cut side only, season and grill for 30 seconds on cut side only. Set aside and let cool, then remove core and chop.

Dry, season and oil the tuna steaks. Place on the hottest part of the grill, and cook for about 2 minutes on each side, leaving the center very rare. Let cool. Using a serrated knife, carefully cut into ½-inch slices.

To Assemble

Divide the romaine on a platter; arrange all the vegetables, and then top with the tuna. Serve with the Roasted Tomato Vinaigrette and garnish with the olives. This salad travels well, if dressed at the last minute.

ARTICHOKE GUACAMOLE

Just like classic guacamole, this condiment goes with everything. Really! Canned artichokes should be a staple in your pantry. They can be used in a multitude of dishes and are robust enough to travel well. Buying hearts or quarters means that someone else has done all the hard work for you!

Makes approximately 3 cups

1 12 oz can artichoke hearts, drained and chopped

2 jalapeños, stemmed, seeded and minced

1 small red onion, minced

3 Tbsp minced fresh cilantro

2 Roma tomatoes, diced

2 cloves garlic, minced

1 Tbsp chili powder

1 tsp cumin

¼ cup olive oil

1-2 limes, juiced

2 tsp sesame oil

Salt and pepper

Optional, 4 oz cooked bacon, chopped

In a medium mixing bowl, combine all the ingredients. Taste and adjust the lime juice, salt and pepper. Makes approximately 3 cups

Everything's better with bacon! New nutritional trends are even supporting this. A concern may be the preservatives and curing agents. Uncured, natural bacon is now readily available.

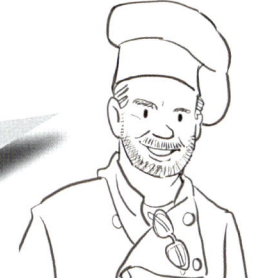

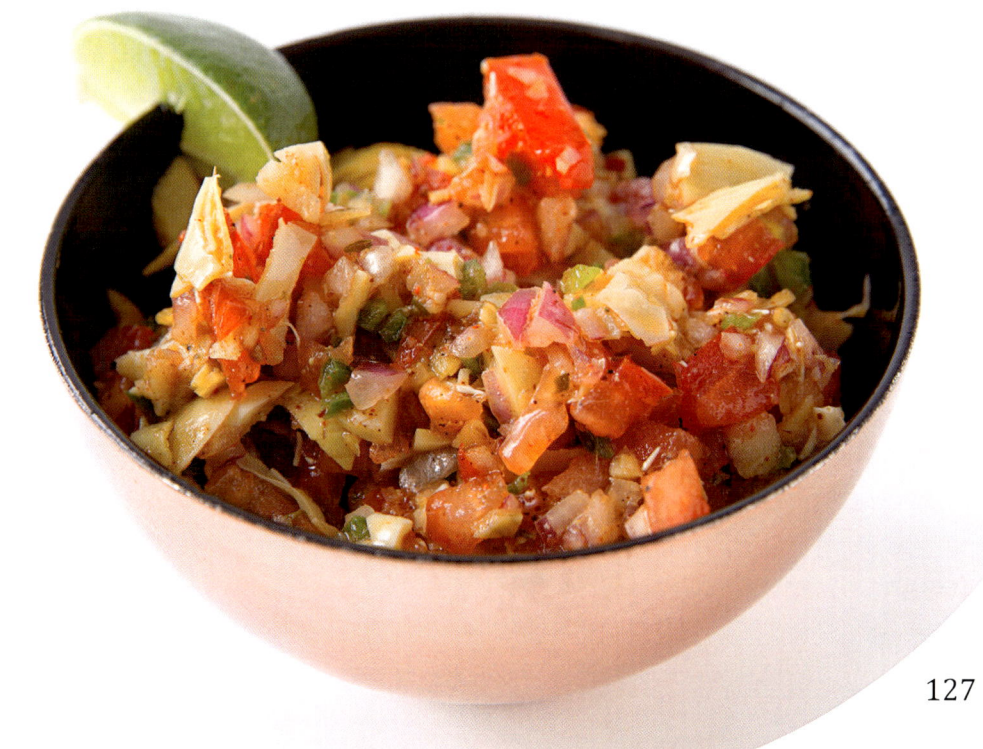

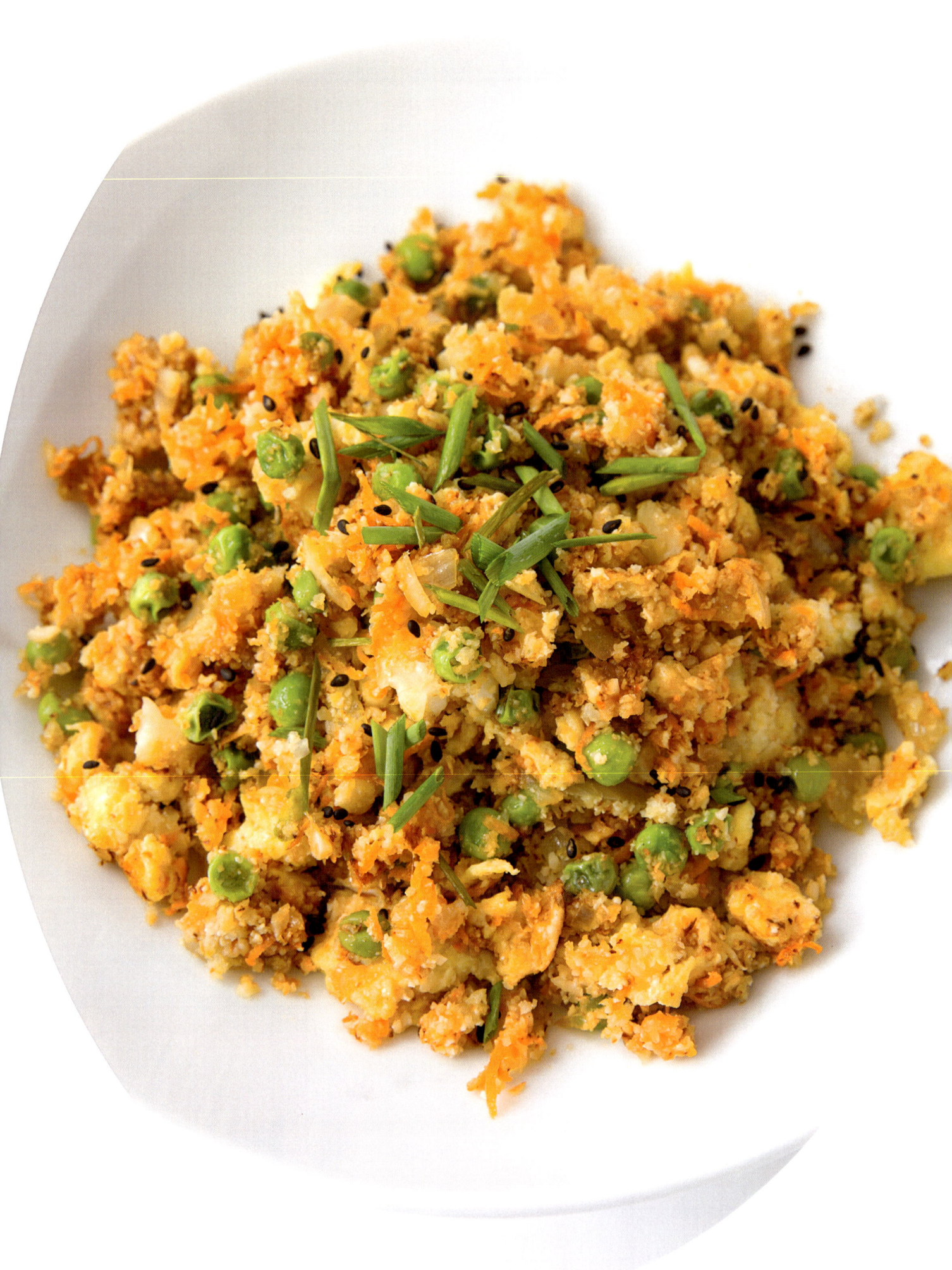

CAULIFLOWER FRIED "RICE"
Makes 4 Servings

3 Tbsp avocado oil, divided

2 eggs, beaten

½ head cauliflower, grated

1 carrot, grated

3-4 garlic cloves, minced

½ cup onion, diced

½ cup frozen peas

3 Tbsp tamari (gluten-free soy sauce)

Heat a small non-stick skillet on medium heat. When hot, add 1 Tbsp oil, then add the eggs. Quickly scramble and when just set, remove and let cool, then chop.

Heat a large skillet on high heat. When hot, add remaining 2 Tbsp oil then the cauliflower and the carrots. Cook for about 2 minutes, and add the garlic and onion. Cook for 2-3 more minutes, or until onions become soft and transparent. Stir in the peas, eggs and tamari and cook for 1-2 minutes until heated through. Serve immediately.

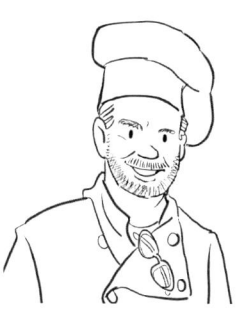

Today, you can purchase all types of prepped vegetables in the supermarket. Although it is easy to make at home, grated cauliflower, also known as cauliflower rice, is a new addition to the freezer section, and can be purchased in most stores.

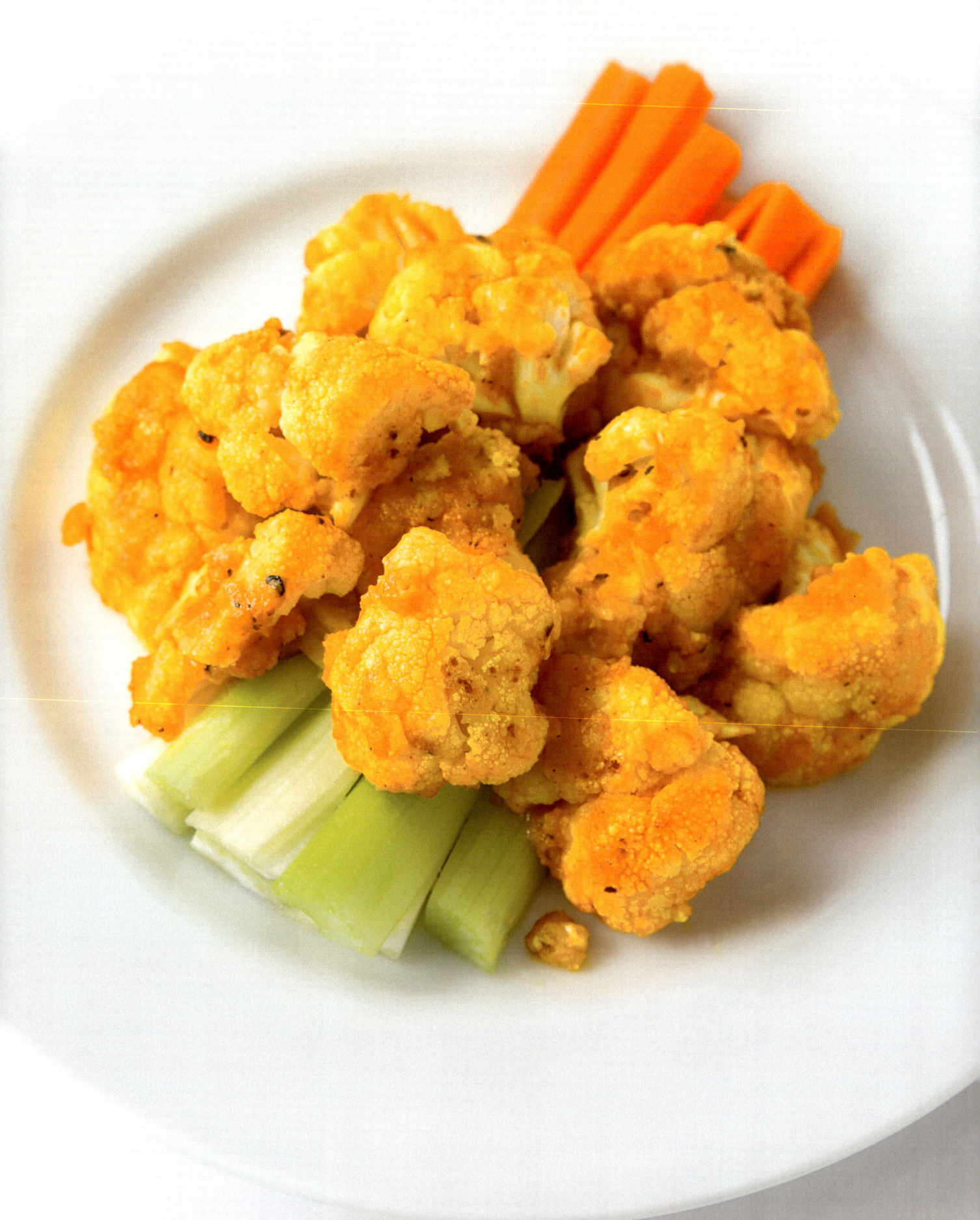

BUFFALO CAULIFLOWER
This is a favorite of Master Will Clark.
Makes 4 Servings

½ cup brown rice flour

½ cup gluten-free breadcrumbs

1 Tbsp garlic powder

1 Tbsp onion powder

1 Tbsp turmeric

1 tsp sea salt

⅓ cup water

1½ lbs cauliflower florets

½ cup hot sauce, such as Durkees

2 Tbsp stemmed and minced Italian parsley

Preheat oven to 450°F.

In a medium mixing bowl, add the flour, breadcrumbs, garlic powder, onion powder, turmeric and sea salt. Whisk in the water. Toss the cauliflower florets in the mixture and place evenly on a parchment lined baking sheet. Cook for 8 minutes then remove from the oven.

Place the cauliflower back in the mixing bowl and toss with hot sauce. Place back on the sheet pan and pop in the oven for 10 minutes. Garnish with parsley leaves. Serve immediately or let cool.

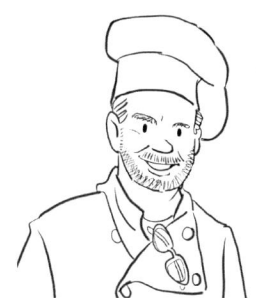

I use gluten-free breadcrumbs for this dish, which adds the desired crunch, without the wheat.

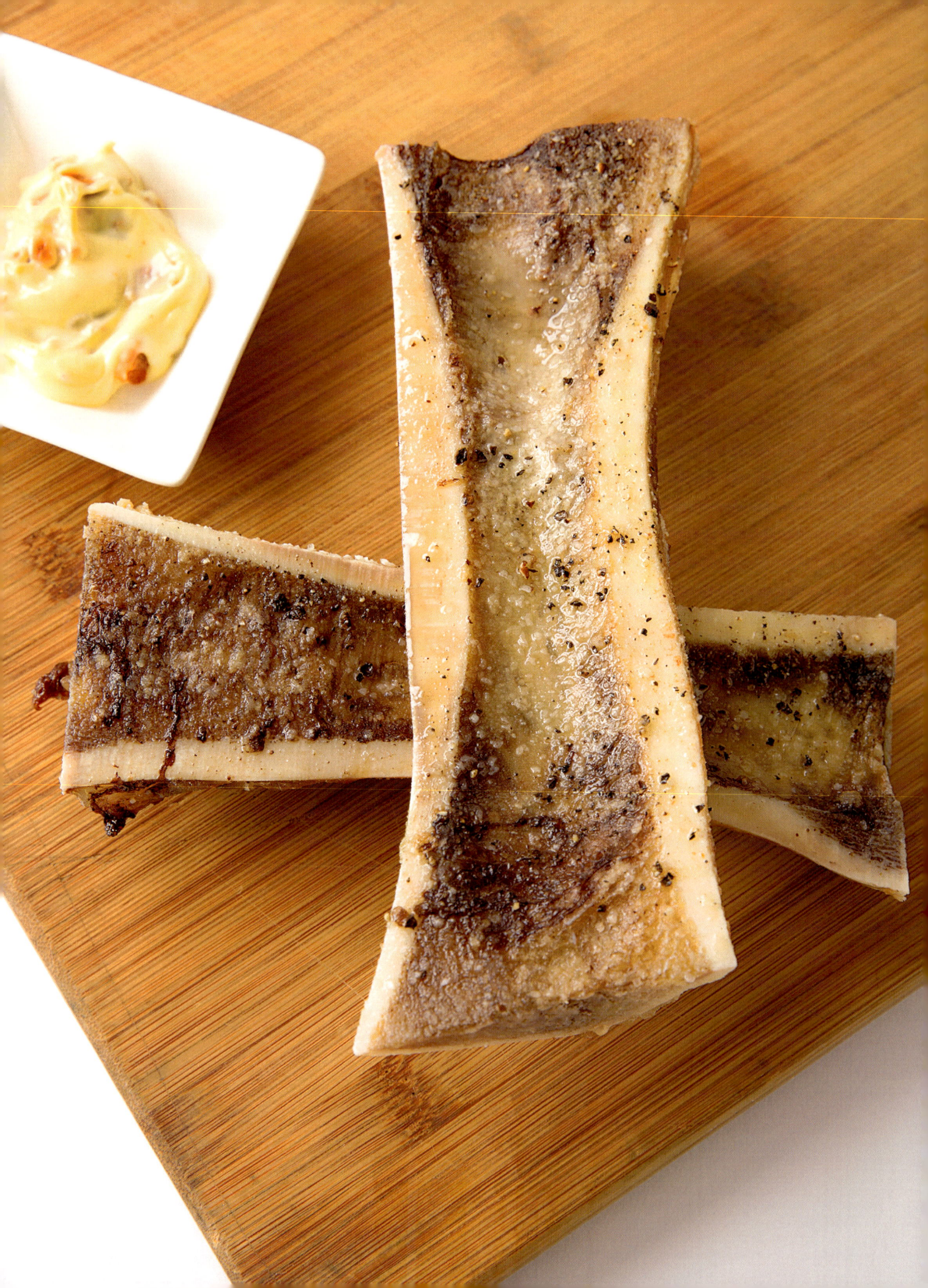

ROASTED MARROW BONES
Bacon Mayonnaise
Makes 4 Servings

> You can find marrow bones split lengthwise very readily in supermarkets, natural food stores and any good butcher shop. This appetizer is so easy and delicious, and although rich and high in fat, it is full of essential nutrients. I call them "canoes." You'll see them often now served in bistro-style restaurants.

Roasted Marrow Bones

2 each beef marrow
   bones, cut in half
   lengthways
1 Tbsp olive oil
Salt and pepper

Preheat oven to 425°F.

Place the marrow bones on a sheet pan, brush with olive oil, then season with salt and pepper. Roast for about 15-20 minutes or until both the bones and marrow are golden brown. Serve immediately.

Bacon Mayonnaise

3 egg yolks
1 Tbsp Dijon mustard
1 Tbsp lemon juice
1 Tbsp white wine
   vinegar
¼ cup liquid bacon fat,
   warm
¼ cup avocado oil
Salt
Tabasco

Whisk together the egg yolks, mustard, lemon juice and vinegar in a medium mixing bowl. While whisking, slowly pour in the bacon fat and avocado oil. Season with salt and Tabasco. Taste and adjust the seasonings. If not using immediately, cover and refrigerate. May be refrigerated up to 3 days. Makes about ¾ cup

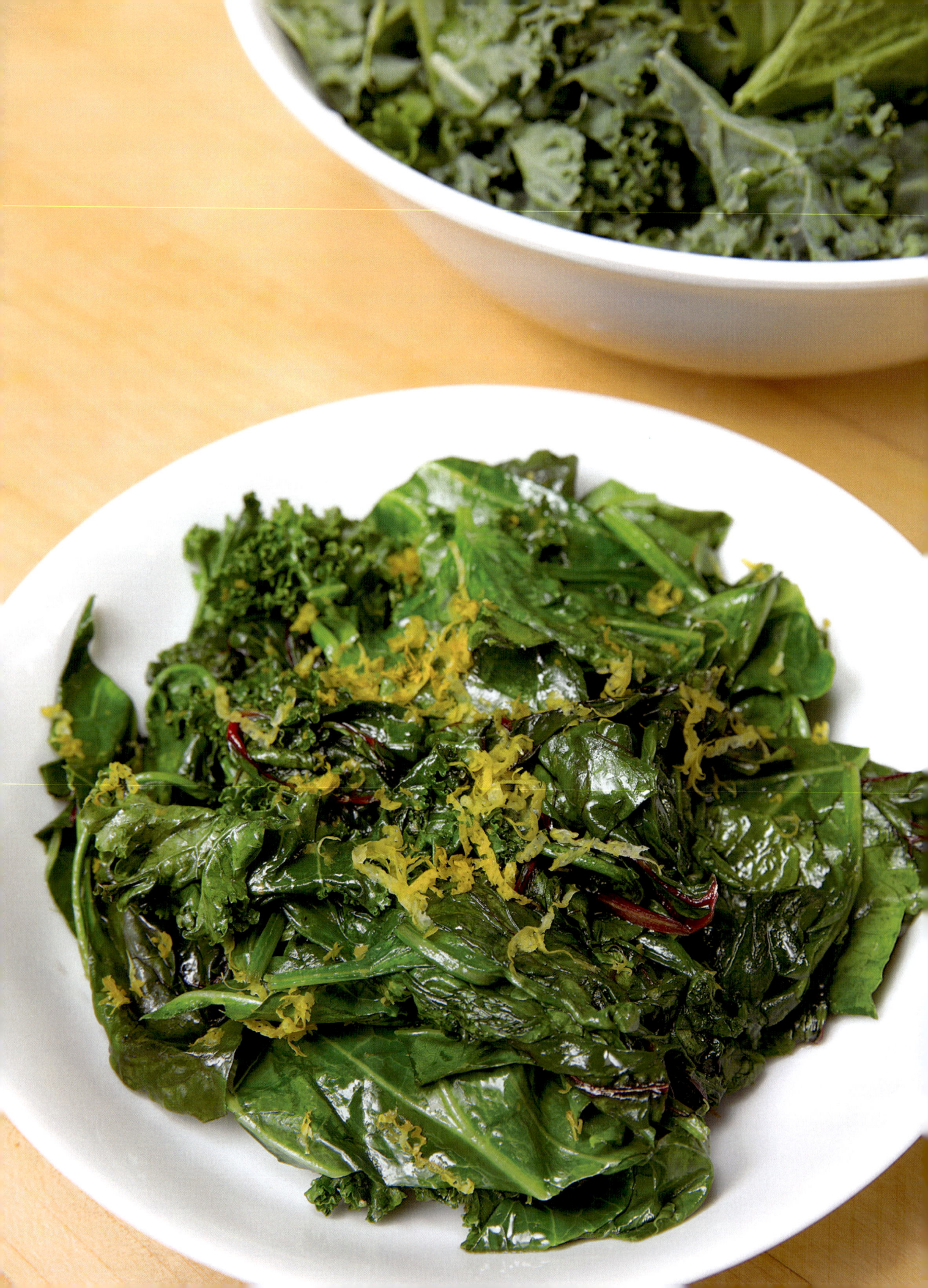

SAUTÉED LEAFY GREENS
You can add this dish to practically any entrée. I incorporate this into my daily power breakfast.
Makes 4 Servings

1 Tbsp olive or avocado oil

8 oz assorted greens, washed

Salt and pepper

Heat a large skillet on medium heat. When hot, add the oil, greens and salt and pepper. Cook, while stirring and turning frequently until the greens are just wilted. Remove and serve immediately.

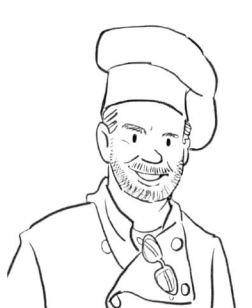

Spinach, kale, arugula, chard, bok choy, mustard greens, collard greens... the list is long. These leafy greens are a fantastic side to any dish, and can be made a regular part of your diet. You can also experiment with different flavorings, such as minced garlic, chopped herbs, lemon juice, pumpkin seeds, etc.

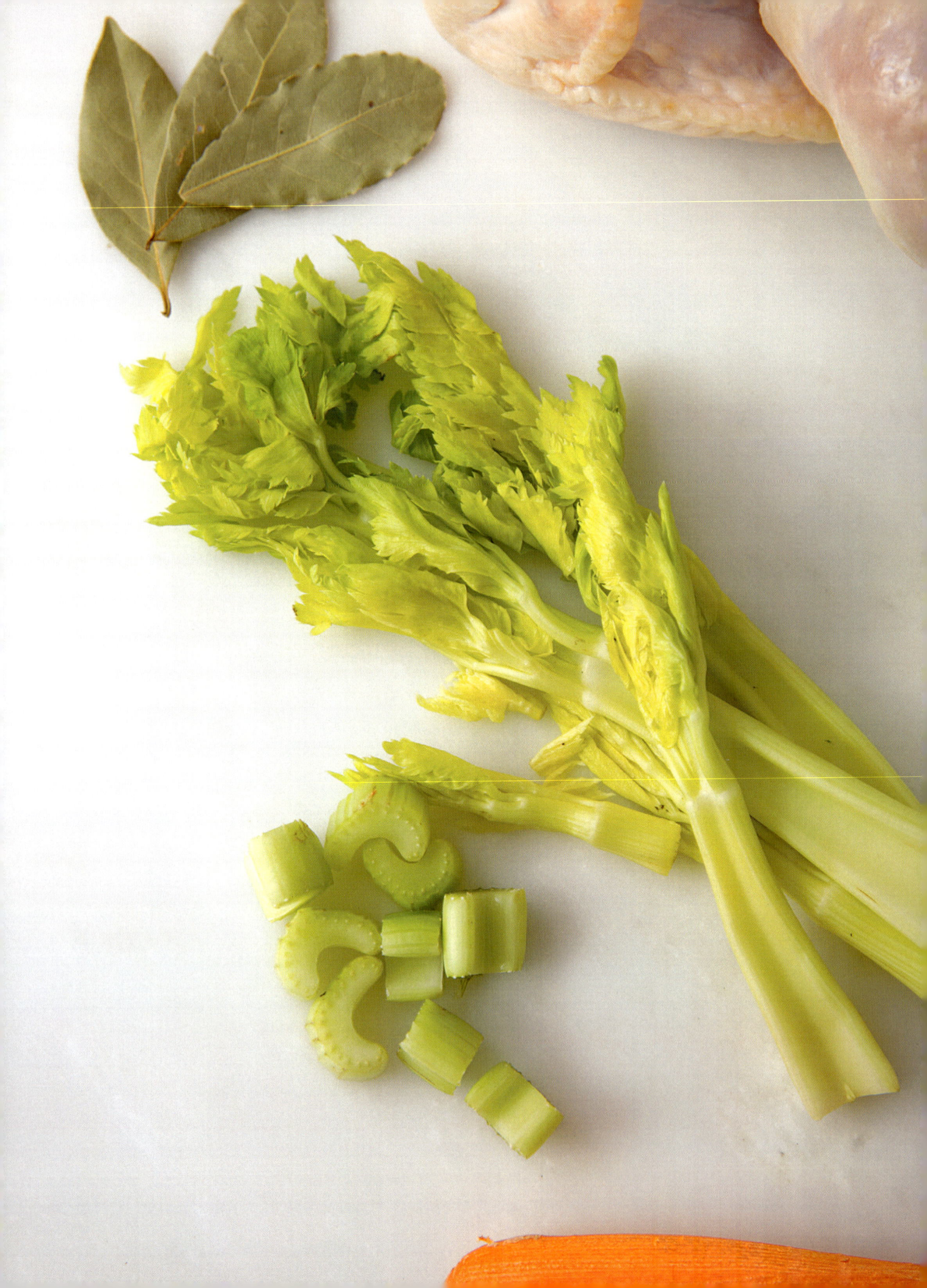

INDEX

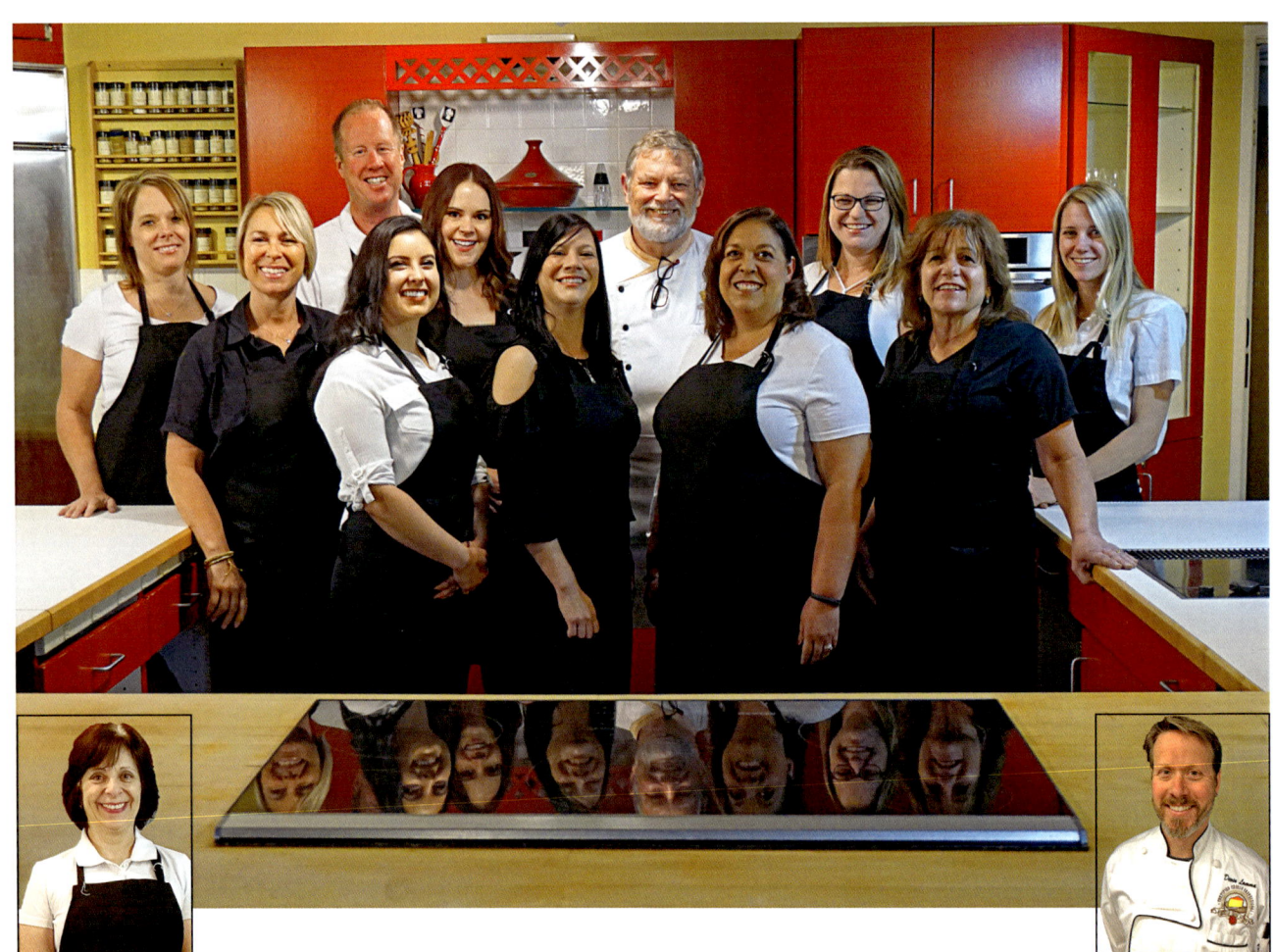

ACKNOWLEDGEMENTS

My first acknowledgement goes to my wonderful wife, Jayne, who was the driving force in launching my second career as a self-employed culinary instructor. She is a constant in my life and has always been there with encouragement to take on the challenges I faced. Her assistance with the writing and production of this book has been invaluable.

I thank Master William Clark, 7th Degree Black Belt in Shaolin Kempo Karate, for his unique wisdom and friendship, and the guidance required in not only constructing this cookbook, but my accomplishments as a martial artist. I also want to thank Janelle Clark for being the first line of review of these recipes.

My thanks go to my amazing staff at The Seasoned Chef Cooking School and The Gourmet Spoon, who not only help provide my students with great culinary learning experiences, but have tested, tasted and critiqued all of these recipes, notably Elsa Elder, Kris Geeting, Kathryn Harper, Devin Lamma, Donna Marrone, Litsa Monsell, Mike O'Rourke, Aarika Ortiz (two fist pumps for grinding it out in the homestretch!), Victoria Partridge, and Jenna Vosburgh and all of my culinary assistants over the last 18 years.

Cathy Harokopis, a great friend and an amazing cook, my appreciation for all of your support through the years and your recipe inspiration.

A special thanks to Katherine D'Souza and Jodie Leschuk, who in addition to managing The Seasoned Chef Cooking School with grace and wisdom, were instrumental in the construction of this cookbook.

To my culinary mentors, Chef Henri Bergmans, Chef Sharon Polster and Chef Darren Denny, I give thanks for all of the great culinary experiences that have been the foundation of my teaching skills.

Many thanks to Susan Stevens, the former owner of The Seasoned Chef Cooking School, who greatly helped me develop my teaching talents and taught me the importance of properly written recipes. To the Colorado Z Ultimate main instructors, past and present, whose lifestyles and good health are the inspiration for this book, with a special nod to Master Emily Carlson and Sensei Anya Adams. With sincere gratitude to Jan McDaniel, Joe McDaniel and Jennifer Olson for holding my hand through the entire production process. Lastly, a special note to Keith Jones and R.J. Harrington, who both hold special places in my life of culinary adventures…

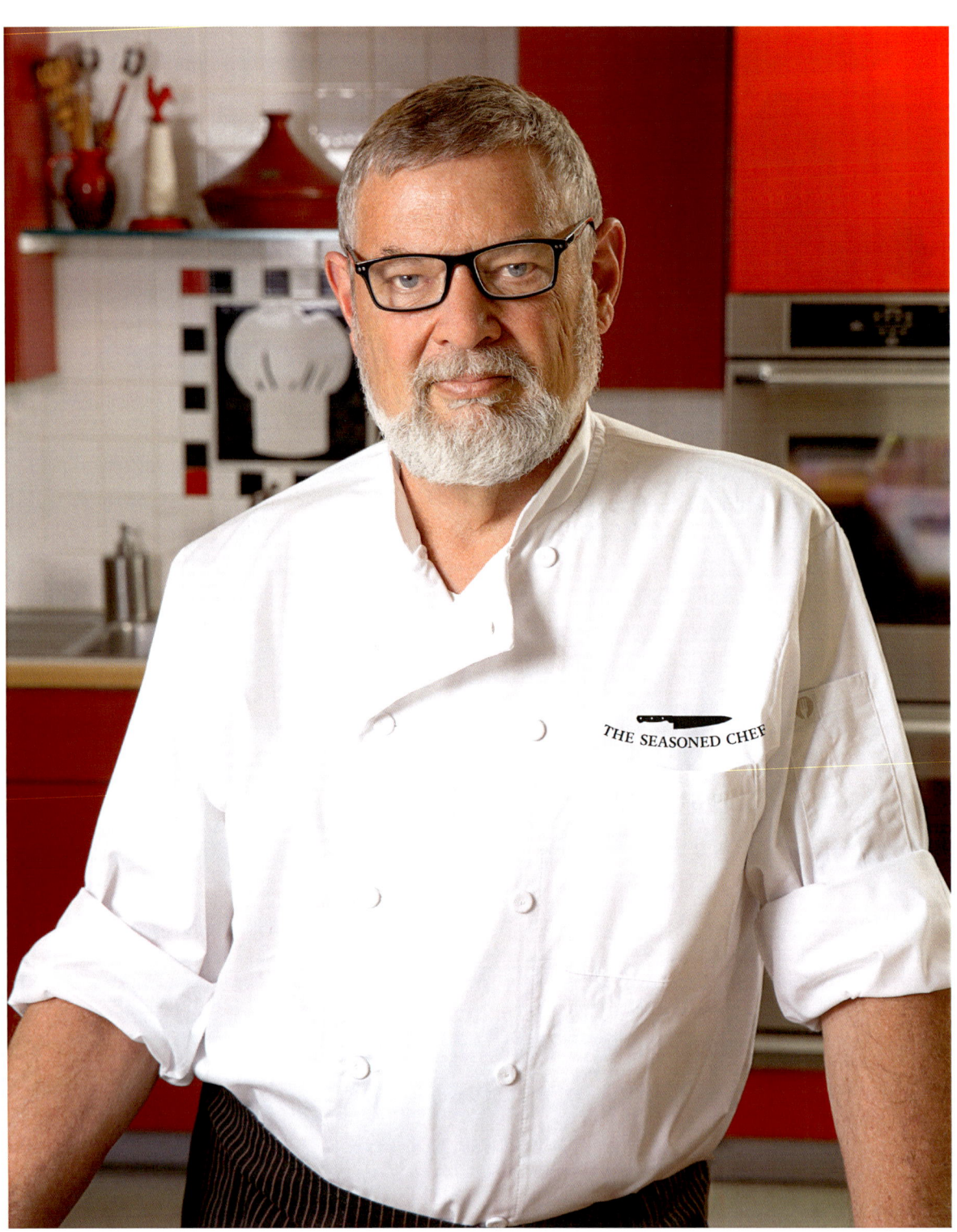

ABOUT THE AUTHOR

Chef Dan Witherspoon is an award-winning, classically-trained chef whose primary passion is teaching home and recreational chefs the fundamentals needed to cook well at home.

After working under acclaimed Belgian chef Henri Bergmans and leading kitchens as an executive chef in both Southern California and Colorado, Chef Dan now focuses his attention towards instruction. As the owner, director, and lead instructor at both The Seasoned Chef Cooking School and The Gourmet Spoon in Denver, Colorado, Chef Dan is widely known for taking the mystery out of the cooking process. In his 37 years of professional cooking experience and 18 years of professional teaching, Chef Dan has been consistently committed to helping students learn to simply, affordably, and quickly make a delicious and healthy meal on their own at home.

Dan is a second-degree black belt in Kempo Karate, training with Z Ultimate self-defense studios. Chef Dan lives in Denver, Colorado, with his wife and continues to teach home and recreational chefs most days in both corporate team building and small group settings. He has recently beaten a rare form of cancer, multiple myeloma, and in addition to the excellent treatment he received from his medical specialists, he credits beating the disease and staying in remission through his diet of fresh vegetables, lean produce, whole grains and good fats. He is living proof that food is more than just fuel, and can be the best defense to maintaining optimum health, wellness and vitality.

More information about Chef Dan can be found on his LinkedIn page www.linkedin.com/in/dan-witherspoon/ or on www.theseasonedchef.com.

LEARN MORE ABOUT US

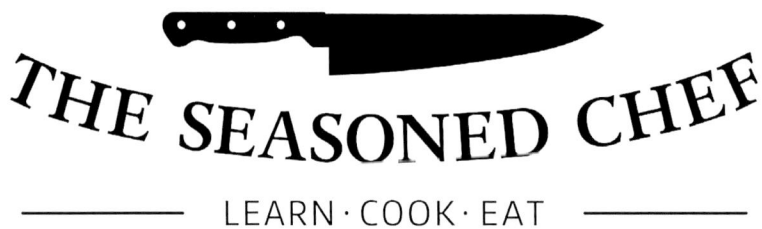

We've been teaching Denver how to cook for over 25 years!

The Seasoned Chef Cooking School
999 Jasmine Street, Suite 100
Denver, CO 80220
303.377.3222
www.theseasonedchef.com

Cooking Classes * Culinary Team Building * Special Events

5280 Magazine Top Cooking School 2006, 2009, 2010
Westword's Best Cooking School 2018

Follow Us!

www.facebook.com/TheSeasonedChef
www.youtube.com/TheSeasonedChef
www.twitter.com/#TheSeasonedChef
www.instagram.com/The Seasoned Chef (@the_seasoned_chef)

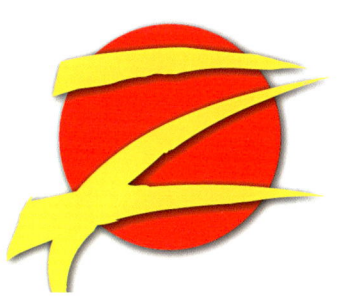